Contested Issues in the Evaluation of Child Sexual Abuse

This book represents a significant contribution to the highly contested debate surrounding how allegations of child sexual abuse should be evaluated. Despite decades of substantial research in this sensitive area, professional consensus remains elusive. A particular source of contention is the sensitivity vs. specificity debate; whether evaluators should give priority to reducing the number of true allegations that are labelled false or to reducing the number of false allegations that are labelled true.

This edited collection aims to address directly and offer new insights into this debate. It responds directly to Kuehnle and Connell's edited volume, *The Evaluation of Child Sexual Abuse Allegations: A Comprehensive Guide to Assessment and Testimony (2009)*, which included chapters which advocated strong specificity positions at the expense of sensitivity. The chapters in this collection feature both challenges to, and replies by, the authors in Kuehnle and Connell's book, making this an essential resource that moves the debate forward.

This book was originally published as a special issue of the *Journal of Child Sexual Abuse*.

Kathleen Coulborn Faller, PhD, A.C.S.W., D.C.S.W., is Marion Elizabeth Blue Professor of Children and Families, University of Michigan, USA, and Director of the Family Assessment Clinic, which evaluates, treats, and provides case record reviews on complex child welfare and sexual abuse cases. She is author of nine books and over 90 research and clinical articles.

Mark D. Everson, PhD, is Professor and Director of the Program on Childhood Trauma and Maltreatment, Department of Psychiatry, University of North Carolina at Chapel Hill, USA. His career has focused on improving the reliability and accuracy of forensic assessments of alleged child abuse.

Contested Issues in the Evaluation of Child Sexual Abuse
A Response to Questions Raised in Kuehnle and Connell's Edited Collection

Edited by
Kathleen Coulborn Faller and Mark D. Everson

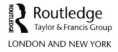

LONDON AND NEW YORK

First published 2014
by Routledge
2 Park Square, Milton Park, Abingdon, Oxon, OX14 4RN, UK

and by Routledge
711 Third Avenue, New York, NY 10017, USA

Routledge is an imprint of the Taylor & Francis Group, an informa business

© 2014 Taylor & Francis

All rights reserved. No part of this book may be reprinted or reproduced or utilised in any form or by any electronic, mechanical, or other means, now known or hereafter invented, including photocopying and recording, or in any information storage or retrieval system, without permission in writing from the publishers.

Trademark notice: Product or corporate names may be trademarks or registered trademarks, and are used only for identification and explanation without intent to infringe.

British Library Cataloguing in Publication Data
A catalogue record for this book is available from the British Library

ISBN13: 978-1-138-77485-8

Typeset in Garamond
by Taylor & Francis Books

Publisher's Note
The publisher accepts responsibility for any inconsistencies that may have arisen during the conversion of this book from journal articles to book chapters, namely the possible inclusion of journal terminology.

Disclaimer
Every effort has been made to contact copyright holders for their permission to reprint material in this book. The publishers would be grateful to hear from any copyright holder who is not here acknowledged and will undertake to rectify any errors or omissions in future editions of this book.

Contents

Citation Information — vii
Notes on Contributors — ix
*Preface: Contested Issues in the Evaluation of Child Sexual Abuse:
A Response to Questions Raised in Kuehnle and Connell's Edited Collection* — xiii

Section 1: Balancing Sensitivity and Specificity in Evaluation of Sexual Abuse

1. Contested Issues in the Evaluation of Child Sexual Abuse Allegations: Why Consensus on Best Practice Remains Elusive
   Kathleen Coulborn Faller and Mark D. Everson — 2

2. Interviewing Children Versus Tossing Coins: Accurately Assessing the Diagnosticity of Children's Disclosures of Abuse
   Thomas D. Lyon, Elizabeth C. Ahern, and Nicholas Scurich — 18

3. Reliability of Professional Judgments in Forensic Child Sexual Abuse Evaluations: Unsettled or Unsettling Science?
   Mark D. Everson, José Miguel Sandoval, Nancy Berson, Mary Crowson, and Harriet Robinson — 44

4. Mental Health Professionals in Children's Advocacy Centers: Is There Role Conflict?
   Theodore P. Cross, Janet E. Fine, Lisa M. Jones, and Wendy A. Walsh — 63

5. Base Rates, Multiple Indicators, and Comprehensive Forensic Evaluations: Why Sexualized Behavior Still Counts in Assessments of Child Sexual Abuse Allegations
   Mark D. Everson and Kathleen Coulborn Faller — 81

6. A Call for Field-Relevant Research about Child Forensic Interviewing for Child Protection
   Erna Olafson — 108

Section 2: Commentaries and Responses

7. "Nobody's Perfect"—Partial Disagreement with Herman, Faust, Bridges, and Ahern
   John E. B. Myers — 130

CONTENTS

8. Comment on Cross, Fine, Jones, and Walsh (2012): Do Mental Health Professionals Who Serve on/with Child Advocacy Centers Experience Role Conflict?
   Colleen Friend — 137

9. Comment on Cross, Fine, Jones, and Walsh (2012): We Are Now on the Same Page
   Seth L. Goldstein — 144

10. Comment on Cross, Fine, Jones, and Walsh (2012): Good Therapeutic Services—Therapeutic Advocacy and Forensic Neutrality
    Mary Connell — 148

11. A Response to Commentary on Faust, Bridges, and Ahern's (2009) "Methods for the Identification of Sexually Abused Children"
    David C. Ahern, Ana J. Bridges, and David Faust — 156

12. What Poole and Wolfe (2009) Actually Said: A Comment on Everson and Faller (2012)
    Debra Ann Poole — 166

Index — 171

Citation Information

The chapters in this book were originally published in the *Journal of Child Sexual Abuse*, volume 21, issue 1 (February 2012) and volume 21, issue 2 (April). When citing this material, please use the original page numbering for each article, as follows:

Chapter 1
Contested Issues in the Evaluation of Child Sexual Abuse Allegations: Why Consensus on Best Practice Remains Elusive
Kathleen Coulborn Faller and Mark D. Everson
Journal of Child Sexual Abuse, volume 21, issue 1 (February 2012) pp. 3-18

Chapter 2
Interviewing Children Versus Tossing Coins: Accurately Assessing the Diagnosticity of Children's Disclosures of Abuse
Thomas D. Lyon, Elizabeth C. Ahern, and Nicholas Scurich
Journal of Child Sexual Abuse, volume 21, issue 1 (February 2012) pp. 19-44

Chapter 3
Reliability of Professional Judgments in Forensic Child Sexual Abuse Evaluations: Unsettled or Unsettling Science?
Mark D. Everson, José Miguel Sandoval, Nancy Berson, Mary Crowson, and Harriet Robinson
Journal of Child Sexual Abuse, volume 21, issue 1 (February 2012) pp. 72-90

Chapter 4
Mental Health Professionals in Children's Advocacy Centers: Is There Role Conflict?
Theodore P. Cross, Janet E. Fine, Lisa M. Jones, and Wendy A. Walsh
Journal of Child Sexual Abuse, volume 21, issue 1 (February 2012) pp. 91-108

Chapter 5
Base Rates, Multiple Indicators, and Comprehensive Forensic Evaluations: Why Sexualized Behavior Still Counts in Assessments of Child Sexual Abuse Allegations
Mark D. Everson and Kathleen Coulborn Faller
Journal of Child Sexual Abuse, volume 21, issue 1 (February 2012) pp. 45-71

Chapter 6
A Call for Field-Relevant Research about Child Forensic Interviewing for Child Protection

Erna Olafson
Journal of Child Sexual Abuse, volume 21, issue 1 (February 2012) pp. 109-129

Chapter 7
"Nobody's Perfect"—Partial Disagreement with Herman, Faust, Bridges, and Ahern
John E. B. Myers
Journal of Child Sexual Abuse, volume 21, issue 2 (April) pp. 203-209

Chapter 8
Comment on Cross, Fine, Jones, and Walsh (2012): Do Mental Health Professionals Who Serve on/with Child Advocacy Centers Experience Role Conflict?
Colleen Friend
Journal of Child Sexual Abuse, volume 21, issue 2 (April) pp. 233-239

Chapter 9
Comment on Cross, Fine, Jones, and Walsh (2012): We Are Now on the Same Page
Seth L. Goldstein
Journal of Child Sexual Abuse, volume 21, issue 2 (April) pp. 240-243

Chapter 10
Comment on Cross, Fine, Jones, and Walsh (2012): Good Therapeutic Services—Therapeutic Advocacy and Forensic Neutrality
Mary Connell
Journal of Child Sexual Abuse, volume 21, issue 2 (April) pp. 225-232

Chapter 11
A Response to Commentary on Faust, Bridges, and Ahern's (2009) "Methods for the Identification of Sexually Abused Children"
David C. Ahern, Ana J. Bridges, and David Faust
Journal of Child Sexual Abuse, volume 21, issue 2 (April) pp. 210-219

Chapter 12
What Poole and Wolfe (2009) Actually Said: A Comment on Everson and Faller (2012)
Debra Ann Poole
Journal of Child Sexual Abuse, volume 21, issue 2 (April) pp. 220-224

Please direct any queries you may have about the citations to clsuk.permissions@cengage.com

Notes on Contributors

David C. Ahern, PhD, Alpert Medical School of Brown University, Providence, RI, USA.

Elizabeth C. Ahern, MA, is a PhD candidate in developmental psychology at the University of Southern California, USA. She researches children's disclosure of maltreatment, truth induction methods, and emergent lie-telling ability. She is also a child interviewing specialist and conducts training on child interviewing.

Nancy Berson, LCSW, is Assistant Director of the Program on Childhood Trauma and Maltreatment at the University of North Carolina at Chapel Hill, USA. She has had more than 30 years of experience in working with abused and neglected children, including coordinating the Duke University Child Protection Team and working with the Guardian ad Litem Program and Departments of Social Services.

Ana J. Bridges, PhD, Department of Psychology, University of Arkansas, Fayetteville, AR, USA.

Mary Connell, EdD, Independent Practice, Fort Worth, Texas, USA.

Theodore P. Cross is a research full professor at the Children and Family Research Center in the School of Social Work at the University of Illinois at Urbana-Champaign, USA. He directed the Multisite Evaluation of Children's Advocacy Centers and has published numerous studies for more than 21 years on the investigation and response to child abuse.

Mary Crowson, PhD, provides psychological services to maltreated children and their caregivers. Her clinical work at the University of North Carolina includes interventions for very young children who have been maltreated, psychological evaluations of children with histories of maltreatment, and expert testimony and consultation regarding child abuse disclosures and the impact of abuse.

Mark D. Everson, PhD, is Professor and Director of the Program on Childhood Trauma and Maltreatment, Department of Psychiatry, University of North Carolina at Chapel Hill, USA. His career has focused on improving the reliability and accuracy of forensic assessments of alleged child abuse.

Kathleen Coulborn Faller, PhD, A.C.S.W., D.C.S.W., is Marion Elizabeth Blue Professor of Children and Families, University of Michigan, USA, and Director of the Family Assessment Clinic, which evaluates, treats, and provides case record reviews on complex child welfare and sexual abuse cases. She is author of nine books and over 90 research and clinical articles.

Janet E. Fine, MS, is the executive director of the Massachusetts Office for Victim Assistance and for the past 28 years has been a leader in victim rights and services and the development of multidisciplinary teams and Children's Advocacy Centers (CAC). She was a founder of two CACs in Massachusetts and the Massachusetts Children's Alliance, chaired the committee that created the national standards for CACs, and currently serves on the National Children's Alliance Board.

David Faust, PhD, Department of Psychology, University of Rhode Island, Kingston, RI, and Alpert Medical School of Brown University, Providence, RI, USA.

Colleen Friend, PhD, LCSW, is the director of the CSULA Child Sexual Abuse and Family Violence Institute in Los Angeles, California, USA. She was the past director of both the Los Angeles County Child Abuse Crisis Center and Stuart House.

Seth L. Goldstein, Esq., is a California attorney in private practice handling child abuse cases in the civil, family law and juvenile courts. He also represents mental health professionals in licensing and discipline matters. He was also a law enforcement officer, serving as a co-chairman of an early multidisciplinary team. He is the author of *The Sexual Exploitation of Children: A Practical Guide to Assessment, Investigation and Intervention* (1999).

Lisa M. Jones, PhD, is a research associate professor of psychology at the Crimes Against Children Research Center at the University of New Hampshire, USA. She has been conducting research on issues of child victimization intervention and prevention for more than 10 years, including research on CACs, child maltreatment trends, children's experiences with sexual abuse investigations, and Internet crimes against children.

Thomas D. Lyon, PhD, JD, is the Judge Edward J. and Ruey L. Guirado Chair in Law and Psychology at the University of Southern California, USA, and researches child abuse and neglect, child witnesses, and domestic violence. He is the past-president of the American Psychological Association's Section on Child Maltreatment (Division 37) and a former member of the board of directors of the American Professional Society on the Abuse of Children.

John E. B. Myers, JD, is a professor of law at the University of the Pacific, McGeorge School of Law in Sacramento, California, USA.

Erna Olafson, PhD, PsyD, is associate professor of clinical psychiatry and pediatrics at Cincinnati Children's Hospital Medical Center and the University of Cincinnati College of Medicine, USA. She has directed the Cincinnati Children's Hospital Childhood Trust Child Forensic Training Program since 1999.

Debra Ann Poole, Department of Psychology, Central Michigan University, Mt. Pleasant, Michigan, USA.

Harriet Robinson, MSW, LCSW, currently serves as case manager in the University of North Carolina Hospital's Emergency Medicine Department, USA. Formerly she provided clinical and forensic services at the University of North Carolina Program on Childhood Trauma and Maltreatment.

NOTES ON CONTRIBUTORS

José Miguel Sandoval, MSc, MPhil, is a guest lecturer in statistics at the Duke University Center for International Development, USA. Formerly he served as a statistician at the University of North Carolina Injury Prevention Research Center and at the Duke University Center on Child and Family Policy.

Nicholas Scurich, MA, is a PhD candidate in quantitative psychology at the University of Southern California, USA. He studies normative and descriptive models of juridical decision making.

Wendy A. Walsh, PhD, is a research associate professor of sociology at the Crimes Against Children Research Center at the University of New Hampshire, USA. She conducts applied research on the system response to child maltreatment, including Children's Advocacy Centers, access to services for victims, and criminal justice outcomes.

Contested Issues in the Evaluation of Child Sexual Abuse: A Response to Questions Raised in Kuehnle and Connell's Edited Collection

Child sexual abuse is a violation of trust, a traumatizing event, and a crime. Professionals who are charged with determining whether an allegation of sexual abuse is true bear a heavy burden. The burden is compounded because it is rare to know with certainty whether the allegation is true or false; sexual abuse is usually shrouded in secrecy. The burden is also compounded because of the enormity of normative transgression. The stakes are high for the child, for the accused, and also for the professional evaluating the allegation. Despite over 30 years of practice and research into child sexual abuse, consensus on best practice for evaluating allegations continues to elude professionals, and many issues remain contested.

In this book, we address a number of the contested issues in evaluating child sexual abuse. Some issues relate to evidence from the child: the relevance of children's sexualized behavior in assessing allegations of sexual abuse, the probative value of children's disclosures in determining the likelihood of sexual abuse, and whether sexual abuse should only be substantiated when there is medical or physical evidence or an offender confession. Other issues relate to professional roles: the reliability of professional judgment about the likelihood of sexual abuse, whether it is ethical for a mental health professional to offer an opinion about the likelihood of sexual abuse, and whether there is a conflict of interest for a psychologist to serve as a member of a multidisciplinary team at a Children's Advocacy Center. Finally, relevant research and its interpretation are themes in all of the chapters and all of the commentaries in this volume.

Many of the contested issues derive from differing views about the relative importance of sensitivity – correctly identifying true victims of child sexual abuse (avoiding false negatives), and specificity – correctly identifying false allegations (avoiding false positives). This volume is a response to Kuehnle and Connell's edited book, *The Evaluation of Child Sexual Abuse Allegations: A Comprehensive Guide to Assessment and Testimony*. The interdisciplinary group of professionals comprising the authors of *Contested Issues in the Evaluation of Child Sexual Abuse* believe several of the chapters in Kuehnle and Connell's book err too much on the side of specificity. The authors argue for a balance between sensitivity and specificity. Their critiques of specific chapters in the Kuehnle and Connell book as well as the replies by the Kuehnle and Connell chapter authors initially appeared in the first two issues of volume 21 (2012) of the *Journal of Child Sexual Abuse*. Two years later, the contested issues remain unresolved. The editors of *Contested Issues in the Evaluation of Child Sexual Abuse* are interested in moving forward the debate on the importance of sensitivity and specificity in child sexual abuse evaluation, which we think has the potential to achieve consensus on best practice.

Section 1:

Balancing Sensitivity and Specificity in Evaluation of Sexual Abuse

INTRODUCTION

Contested Issues in the Evaluation of Child Sexual Abuse Allegations: Why Consensus on Best Practice Remains Elusive

KATHLEEN COULBORN FALLER
University of Michigan, Ann Arbor, Michigan, USA

MARK D. EVERSON
University of North Carolina at Chapel Hill, Chapel Hill, North Carolina, USA

This is an introductory article to a special issue of the Journal of Childhood Sexual Abuse *that responds to challenges to current forensic evaluation practice found in Kuehnle and Connell's edited volume* The Evaluation of Child Sexual Abuse Allegations: A Comprehensive Guide to Assessment and Testimony *(2009). This article describes the topics that will be addressed in this issue, summarizes the contents of the Kuehnle and Connell book, and provides a hypothetical case to illustrate potential problems in applying certain perspectives and guidelines offered in the book to actual forensic practice.*

Sometimes unintended consequences are more valuable than intended consequences. Such is the case, we believe, for a recent edited volume by Kathryn Kuehnle and Mary Connell, *The Evaluation of Child Sexual Abuse*

Allegations: A Comprehensive Guide to Assessment and Testimony (2009). In the preface, the two editors succinctly describe as their objective to assist child forensic evaluators in improving their practice. Toward this end, Kuehnle and Connell assembled a group of noted experts from a variety of relevant specialties to share their perspectives on the assessment of child sexual abuse allegations. Many forensic evaluators approach such a book as an opportunity to compare the assessment methodology they use in their everyday practice against the latest recommendations from the experts. Their goal is to update their current "good practice" to best practice standards. An evaluator seeking such assistance from the Kuehnle and Connell book may be dismayed and discouraged. Several chapters in the Kuehnle and Connell volume challenge, if not condemn, the validity of established forensic methodology—the very methodology likely employed by the evaluator. The book raises questions about the acceptability of what has long been considered to be appropriate practice. From the forensic evaluator's perspective, the goal posts marking best practice have not merely been shifted. Shifting is expected. They have been moved to a different field altogether.

One chapter of the book, for example, describes current forensic practice as relying primarily on "unverified methods or conjecture" and on "unwarranted practices" (Faust, Bridges, & Ahern, 2009a, p. 4). A second chapter criticizes previous research on behavior indicators of abuse as seriously flawed, thereby casting doubt on much known about the symptoms differentiating sexually abused from nonabused children (Bridges, Faust, & Ahern, 2009). This chapter is complemented by a third chapter that raises concerns about the reliability and validity of all behavioral symptoms, especially sexualized behavior, in child sexual abuse evaluations (Poole & Wolfe, 2009). A fourth chapter raises questions about the objectivity of CSA assessments conducted in child advocacy centers (CACs) because of possible role conflicts (Connell, 2009a). A fifth chapter condemns much of established forensic practice as unethical because of the weight placed on the child's disclosure statement in case decisions (Herman, 2009). This chapter also calls for "drastic reforms" (Herman, 2009, p. 259) in the assessment and adjudication process that include limiting substantiation only to cases with definitive evidence such as diagnostic medical findings.

While such chapters may provoke heated debate, the Kuehnle and Connell book provides an even greater service by shedding light on why, after 30+ years of concerted efforts by practitioners and researchers alike, the field of forensic evaluation does not enjoy greater consensus on best practice. Although several chapters appropriately balance the interests of the alleged child victim and those of the alleged abuser, a consistent theme throughout much of the book is that false positive errors are a greater problem or concern, even at the child protection level, than false negative errors. This theme is most evident in five key chapters on the decision-making process, three of which comprise the opening section of the book

(Bridges et al., 2009; Connell, 2009b; Faust et al., 2009a, 2009b; Herman, 2009). Other chapters (e.g., Klemfuss & Ceci, 2009; Poole and Wolfe, 2009) reinforce this theme. Moreover, it is noteworthy that in a 20-chapter volume describing itself as "a comprehensive guide to assessment and testimony," there is not a single chapter with a comparable emphasis on the problem of false negative errors. On the whole, therefore, the Kuehnle and Connell book clearly places greater emphasis on *specificity* (assuring that children are not mistakenly identified as sexual abuse victims when they are not) than on *sensitivity* (assuring that true victims of sexual abuse are identified and not missed). This specificity emphasis appears to drive much of the book's criticism of current forensic methodology. An analysis of the Kuehnle and Connell book therefore leads us to speculate that a balanced perspective that places an equal premium on both sensitivity (preventing false negatives) and specificity (preventing false positives) is likely a necessary condition for professional consensus on best practice. False positive errors and false negative errors must be viewed as equally objectionable, at least at the child protective services and family court level. Without such balance, there can be little stability in what is considered to be even accepted practice. In the absence of a balanced perspective, promoters of a specificity emphasis and advocates for a sensitivity emphasis are likely to be dissatisfied with the status quo and consequently push for "improvements" in practice. Since sensitivity and specificity are counterbalancing indices of decision accuracy, gains in one are typically achieved only at the expense of the other. Without an effective counterweight, one side or the other dominates with demands for further improvements or "reforms" until a tipping point is reached.

The authors of this special issue of the *Journal of Child Sexual Abuse* counter a number of the challenges to current practice made in the Kuehnle and Connell book while acknowledging that some of these challenges represent legitimate concerns among forensic evaluators and other child-serving professionals. We also argue that accepted practice must include a balance between sensitivity and specificity (Everson & Sandoval, 2011). Indeed, the empirical evidence is clear that unidentified and mistakenly unsubstantiated cases of sexual abuse are likely much more frequent than false substantiations of untrue cases (Cederborg, Lamb, & Laurell, 2007; Hershkowitz et al., 2006; London, Bruck, Ceci, & Shuman, 2005; Sas & Cunningham, 1995; Trocme & Bala, 2005).

WHAT IS IN KUEHNLE AND CONNELL'S *THE EVALUATION OF CHILD SEXUAL ABUSE ALLEGATIONS: A COMPREHENSIVE GUIDE TO ASSESSMENT AND TESTIMONY?*

Kuehnle and Connell's edited volume covers a wide spectrum of issues related to child sexual abuse evaluation. In the preface, the editors speak of "the extraordinary catastrophe" (p. xi) that can result from faulty assessment techniques. In the introduction, Myers (2009) describes the McMartin Preschool case as one such catastrophe. The first three chapters use Bayesian logic and clinical decision research to criticize decision-making in current forensic practice (Bridges, Faust, & Ahern, 2009; Faust et al., 2009a, 2009b). Two of the articles in this issue of *Journal of Child Sexual Abuse* address the assertions in these first three chapters (Everson & Faller, this issue; Lyon, Ahern, & Scurich, this issue). The Kuehnle and Connell volume also includes two chapters that specifically address psychologists' roles (Clark, 2009) and ethics (Koocher, 2009) related to sexual abuse assessment and treatment. A number of the chapters provide summaries of research on normative child development (Klemfuss & Ceci, 2009), normative child sexual behavior (Poole & Wolfe, 2009), children's memory (Klemfuss & Ceci, 2009), including recovered memories (Greenshoot & Tsethlikai, 2009), and children's suggestibility (Harris, Goodman, Augusti, Chae, & Alley, 2009; Malloy & Quas, 2009). There is a section on the child interview itself (Brown & Lamb, 2009; La Rooy, Lamb, & Pipe, 2009), appropriate and inappropriate techniques for interviewing children about sexual abuse (Pipe & Salmon, 2009), and professional decision-making in child sexual abuse cases (Herman, 2009). One chapter is critical of children's advocacy centers, the organizations that coordinate many child sexual abuse investigations in the United States (Connell, 2009a), and one critiques the use of extended assessments with some children (Connell, 2009b). The final section of the volume covers legal issues, including expert testimony about sexual abuse (Shuman & Austin, 2009) and the knowledge of judges and juries about children's reports of sexual abuse (Buck & Warren, 2009). Each chapter has a summary of guidelines in its conclusion.

The National Institutes of Child Health and Human Development (NICHD) Investigative Interview Protocol (Lamb, Hershkowitz, Orbach, & Esplin, 2008) is advocated by three chapters in the Kuehnle and Connell volume (Brown & Lamb, 2009; Connell, 2009a; Herman, 2009). The NICHD protocol is also printed in its entirety as an appendix to the Kuehnle and Connell book. Two articles in this issue of *JCSA* cite the strengths and centrality of the NICHD Protocol to the process of interviewing children about sexual abuse but also suggest additional valid interview practices (Lyon et al., this issue) and domains appropriate for additional child interview research (Olafson, this issue).

SENSITIVITY VS. SPECIFICITY: DOES IT REALLY MATTER?

The following hypothetical case vignette is provided to illustrate the possible impact of privileging specificity over sensitivity, and applying perspectives found in Kuehnle and Connell's edited volume and related writings, to actual practice.

It is important to emphasize that we have no quarrel with the majority of chapters in the Kuehnle and Connell book. Several, we believe, are excellent summaries of the relevant literature. But the overall lack of balance between sensitivity and specificity and the one-sided condemnation of established practice are troubling and potentially harmful to children. It is critical to recognize that one of the potential audiences for an authoritative volume like the Kuehnle and Connell book are members of the judiciary who may mistake the lack of rebuttal or alternative perspectives as evidence that the individual opinions expressed represent consensus or settled science.

Vignette

Emma, age five, is an only child. Her parents were married for five years before they were able to conceive. Her father has a management position in a utility company, and her mother was working part-time as an administrative assistant for a nonprofit. After Emma's birth, her parents began to have disagreements about money and the family's relationship with maternal relatives, whom her father thought were trying to run their lives. The parents entered counseling with a psychologist, but disagreements continued, eventually resulting in an altercation, in which Emma's father slapped her mother in the face causing her lip to bleed. Both parents were shocked that their disagreements had resulted in physical violence and attempted to control their arguments.

However, after Emma's mother was laid off from her job, the disagreements again escalated. Emma's mother began withholding sex from her father, and there was an incident during which he forced sex on her. The parents thought Emma was asleep, but she was not. In fact, she may have seen what happened because their bedroom door was open.

Each parent threatened the other with divorce. The father actually filed, but then withdrew his petition and redoubled his efforts in counseling. Emma began to exhibit symptoms. She had nightmares, wet the bed, was not following directions in kindergarten, hit other children, and on occasion, would put her fingers in her vagina and then lick them. Her parents asked their psychologist if he would see Emma. Their psychologist declined but gave them referrals to other psychologists covered by the father's insurance.

After interviewing two psychologists, the parents agreed on a female psychologist in private practice who seemed warm and objective, but was guided by chapters in Kuehnle and Connell's book and other literature that emphasizes specificity over sensitivity. Both parents signed the consent for Emma's treatment. To the psychologist, the parents described Emma as very smart but as having a lot of difficulty with peers and school. They provided very limited information about their marital problems, only telling Emma's psychologist that they were in counseling to work on their relationship. The psychologist explained that her role was as the child's therapist and that she would give them feedback from time to time. She also mentioned that she was a mandated reporter. She gathered information about Emma from each parent and Emma's kindergarten teacher using the Child Behavior Checklist and Teacher Report Form. Although the parents did not contradict one another in their reports of Emma's competencies and behaviors, only the mother reported Emma putting her fingers in her vagina and licking them. Emma's therapist was mindful of Chapters 1 through 3 by Faust and colleagues (Bridges et al., 2009; Faust et al., 2009a, 2009b) in Kuehnle and Connell's edited volume about base rates of sexual behaviors and the fallacies of overvaluing abuse indicators in clinical work. She also had read Poole and Wolfe's (2009) chapter that points out that there are no sexual behaviors that are found only in sexually abused children. Therefore, she did not put a great deal of weight on the mother's digital penetration and finger licking report. Since most of Emma's problems were related to school and peers, these problems were Emma's psychologist's focus.

After five sessions, during which the psychologist developed good rapport with Emma, Emma said, "I've got something to show you." Emma pulled down her pants, put her fingers in her vagina, and said, "This is where my daddy licks, and then he puts his noodle in." Emma's therapist nodded, suggested Emma pull her pants back up, but asked no questions. She was aware that she was the child's therapist and knew determining whether Emma had been sexually abused was the role of a forensic interviewer or evaluator, as described by Clark in Chapter 4 (Clark, 2009). She also had read Chapter 8 on normative memory development and the child witness (Klemfuss & Ceci, 2009), Chapter 9 on suggestibility (Harris et al., 2009), and Chapter 12 on children's suggestibility, consensus, and contested issues (Malloy & Quas, 2009) in Kuehnle and Connell's book. Because of her specificity bias, Emma's therapist focused upon young children's weaknesses as reporters, even though their ability to accurately recall information, especially with open ended questions, was highlighted in some of these chapters. Being mindful, therefore, of Emma's young age and consequent suggestibility, the therapist did not want to contaminate her memory or account by asking questions or making comments or interpretations. Emma's psychologist changed the topic and soon ended the session.

Emma's mother had brought Emma to the session. Emma's therapist told her mother that she had to suspend treatment for now "because there are concerns about abuse." She admonished Emma's mother not to talk to Emma about abuse because the concerns would be investigated by Child Protective Services (CPS). Emma's psychologist fulfilled her mandated reporter obligation by informing the CPS intake worker that Emma had made concerning disclosures about abuse, possibly by the father. She declined to turn over her treatment notes, explaining that she was fulfilling her reporting obligation but would need both parents to sign a release to turn over her notes.

Despite minimal information, a CPS investigator went to Emma's school the following day to talk to her. The investigator interviewed Emma in the presence of the school social worker, which was the school's policy. Emma ran around the room and said she was late for recess. When asked if anything had happened, she said she had already talked about "what happened." Finally she sat down and pointed to her vaginal area and said, "That's where the noodle went, right there," and then began to poke one finger in and out of her mouth, saying "umm umm." The investigator decided that there was enough information to have Emma interviewed at the Children's Advocacy Center (CAC). She went to the family home and spoke to Emma's mother, telling her what Emma had said and done in the interview. Since Emma's psychologist had indicated "possibly the father," the CPS investigator advised Emma's mother not to leave Emma alone with her father, but also told her not question Emma. The CAC interview and medical examination were scheduled for a few days later.

During the few days before the CAC visit, Emma's therapist received urgent calls from both parents asking what was going on. The psychologist told them to wait until after the CAC interview. She did not want to interfere with the investigation. The CPS investigator also called the psychologist asking for her treatment notes. The psychologist said she would get the parents' forms for permission to release the notes. Mother gave her permission, but father did not. Since both parents had agreed to treatment, she felt she could not release the notes without the father's agreement. Emma's therapist also learned from the CPS investigator that the CAC used the NICHD protocol. She was relieved and impressed because she knew from reading Chapter 13 (Brown & Lamb, 2009) in Kuehnle and Connell's book and other reading that the NICHD protocol was the most researched protocol and had been demonstrated to elicit more abuse-related information and details, using more open-ended questions, than interviews that did not use the NICHD protocol.

It was a tense few days for Emma's family. Emma asked her mother several times what was wrong, and her mother said, "I'm not supposed to talk about it." Her mother caught Emma sticking her fingers in her vagina again. Her mother scolded Emma, telling her "nice girls don't do that," and Emma said, "Daddy does." Her mother called Emma's therapist again to ask what to do and was again told to wait for the CAC interview. Emma's mother decided to leave the marital home with Emma and go to her mother's for the weekend. She left a note for her husband. The following Monday, Emma's father refiled for divorce, asking for custody and alleging that his wife was making a false accusation of sexual abuse against him.

Tuesday was the CAC interview and medical examination. Emma's interviewer, a father of two, was respected, experienced, and had attended training on the NICHD protocol. Emma was brought by her mother but encountered her father in the parking lot. As is common with CACs, the father (the alleged offender) was not allowed in the building.

Behind the one-way mirror were the CPS investigator, a police officer, and an assistant prosecutor. Emma allowed the interviewer to take her into the interview room and listened as he explained his role and gave her the ground rules. However, she guessed when asked the practice question, "What is my (interviewer's) dog's name?" (The question is intended to inoculate the child against guessing). When asked to tell the interviewer the reason she was talking to him, she said, "I don't know." The interviewer went carefully through the list of probes in the NICHD protocol that were appropriate given the limited information he had from Emma's earlier disclosures. Emma only provided information that her mommy and daddy "fighted" and she did not know what they fought about. The interview was inconclusive. On exam, there were no medical findings, despite Emma's demonstration and statement to her psychologist that the "noodle went in."

When Emma's mother called Emma's psychologist and reported the results of the CAC visit, the psychologist, mindful of Herman's chapter (2009) describing the dangerousness of substantiating a sexual abuse case when there is no "hard evidence," was skeptical about the allegation. From having read Chapter 13 (Brown & Lamb, 2009) in Kuehnle and Connell's edited volume, she knew that approximately two-thirds of children in a large Israeli study (Hershkowitz, Horowitz, & Lamb, 2005) and three-fourths of children in a smaller American study (Pipe et al., 2007) revealed abuse when interviewed using the NICHD protocol. Although she knew that younger children and children whose alleged offender was a family member were less likely to disclose, she was unaware that the percentage of girls ages three to six who made disclosures in the Israeli study when the alleged offender was a parent was about 15% (Hershkowitz et al., 2005). These findings are not included in Brown and Lamb's chapter.

Because of the lack of information from Emma's interview, the multidisciplinary team (MDT), which makes case management decisions at the CAC, invited Emma's therapist to their meeting about Emma's case. Being aware of Connell's Chapter 17 in Kuehnle and Connell proposing role conflict for psychologists working with CACs because of their prosecutorial role, she declined to attend the meeting. Especially given her therapeutic role with Emma, she thought her participation would open her up to ethical challenge, possibly a grievance, and maybe even a lawsuit.

Because findings were sparse and Emma was considered not competent to testify, as often happens with young children, law enforcement and the prosecutor did not pursue the case. The MDT at the CAC recommended an extended forensic evaluation to Emma's mother, one of the services offered by the CAC. Emma's mother called Emma's therapist to ask her advice about the extended forensic evaluation. The therapist had read Chapter 18 in Kuehnle and Connell (Connell, 2009b), which outlines numerous reservations about extended forensic evaluations. For example, guidelines at the end of this chapter point out that extended forensic evaluations are not recorded, they do not have a structured format, there is no formal requirement for the consideration of alternative hypotheses, and there are no clear guidelines about the final report. Emma's therapist cautioned the mother about involving her daughter in the extended assessment process.

Mother followed the therapist's advice about the extended assessment but asked for Emma to return to treatment. Emma's symptoms had worsened after the CAC visit and her parents' separation. Unfortunately, by this time the parents were locked in contentious divorce and custody proceedings. The father refused to agree to have Emma return to therapy with the psychologist because he blamed her for accusing him of sexually abusing his daughter.

This case example highlights potential consequences for children when mental health professionals place greater weight on specificity than sensitivity. Emma's psychologist put no weight on her mother's report of a sexualized behavior, a high probability indicator of sexual abuse (Friedrich, 1999). When Emma made a spontaneous disclosure of sexual abuse by her father to the psychologist and demonstrated advanced sexual knowledge, another high probability indicator (Brilleslijper-Kater, Friedrich, & Corwin, 2004), the psychologist did not follow up with the child (Kuehnle & Connell, 2010). The psychologist felt she needed to suspend treatment because the role of a therapist should be differentiated from that of a child abuse investigator. Moreover, she did not appreciate the importance of her relationship with Emma in prompting Emma's disclosure; this was overshadowed by her concern about Emma's suggestibility and fear of contaminating of Emma's account. The psychologist fulfilled her mandated reporting responsibility in a minimal way, thereby choosing not to share compelling information with investigators.

Like many young children who are sexually abused, Emma made a spontaneous disclosure to someone she trusted but later provided minimal information to strangers, in part because of her experience with family distress and dissolution after disclosure. Being generally cautious and skeptical about sexual abuse reports by young children, the psychologist interpreted the nondisclosure and lack of medical findings to mean the child's report to her was false. She was also mindful of Kuehnle and Connell's (2010) position that a judge or jury determine "the legal truth" (p. 555) of sexual abuse. She was unaware of what a small proportion of three- to six-year-old girls disclose when the offender is a parent and the small proportion of sexually abused children with medical findings (Adams, Harper, Knudson, & Revilla, 1994). Putting greater weight on her professional well-being than on Emma's, she declined requests to be involved in the decision-making process at the CAC. Because of concerns about the lack of empirical support for extended evaluations, she advised Emma's mother against an extended assessment. Emma is left unsafe and struggling on her own to make meaning of her sexual abuse and consequences of disclosure. Regardless of the actions and decisions of Emma's therapist, there will likely be no "happily ever after" for Emma, but her safety could have been assured and services to help her heal made more available had the psychologist followed a different approach. We use this hypothetical case example to contextualize the issues to be addressed in the articles in this special issue of *JCSA*.

ARTICLES IN THIS ISSUE OF *JOURNAL OF CHILD SEXUAL ABUSE*

In addition to this introduction, this issue of the *Journal of Child Sexual Abuse* provides five articles. In the article titled "Interviewing Children Versus Tossing Coins: Accurately Assessing the Diagnosticity of Children's Disclosures of Abuse," Lyon, Ahern, and Scurich assist the reader by providing a "plain English" rendition of Bayesian thinking about probabilities, which formed the basis for Faust and colleagues' criticisms of the diagnostic value of sexual abuse indicators (Bridges et al., 2009; Faust et al., 2009a, 2009b). Lyon and colleagues dispute Faust and colleagues' conclusion that screening criteria for sexual abuse are of little diagnostic value, arguing Faust and colleagues underestimate the likelihood that children seen for sexual abuse assessment have been abused. Lyon and colleagues describe the importance of children's disclosures of sexual abuse, noting that this importance varies depending on the child's age and how the disclosure information was elicited. They also take issue with Herman's (2009) skepticism about the utility of children's disclosures absent "hard evidence," an issue also addressed in the article by Everson and colleagues (this issue). Finally, Lyon and colleagues describe evidence-based strategies, in addition to those found in the NICHD protocol, which can improve the quality of information obtained from children during forensic interviews.

"Base Rates, Multiple Indicators, and Comprehensive Forensic Evaluations: Why Sexualized Behavior Still Counts in Assessments of Child Sexual Abuse Allegations" by Everson and Faller also challenges the first three chapters in Kuehnle and Connell by Faust and colleagues as well as the chapter by Poole and Wolfe. The Everson and Faller article focuses on the varying roles that developmentally inappropriate sexualized behavior may play in the assessment process. They address several concerns or objections that Faust and colleagues and Poole and Wolfe voice about the diagnostic value of sexualized behavior in forensic evaluations. Everson and Faller draw on the pioneering work of the late William Friedrich (Friedrich, 1993, 1999, 2002; Friedrich et al., 2001), who developed the Child Sexual Behavior Inventory (CSBI) and who, using the CSBI, spearheaded research in the United States and other countries that provides estimates of base rates for various sexual behaviors in children with and without histories of sexual abuse. This article also describes the CHIC evaluation model (comprehensive, hypothesis-testing, idiographic, corroborative) as a best practices approach that addresses common criticisms of forensic practice, including the use of sexualized behavior as a possible marker for abuse.

In "Reliability of Professional Judgments in Forensic Child Sexual Abuse Evaluations: Unsettled or Unsettling Science?", Everson, Sandoval, Berson, Crowson, and Robinson take issue with Chapter 11, "Forensic Child Sexual Abuse Evaluations: Accuracy, Ethics, and Admissibility" (Herman, 2009), which asserts that clinical substantiation decisions are unreliable and therefore invalid and unethical. Herman differentiates between "hard" evidence (e.g., conclusive medical evidence or physical evidence; for example, videos of abuse or suspect's confession) and "soft" evidence (e.g., children's statements and behaviors). Taking an extreme specificity-over-sensitivity position, Herman opines that child sexual abuse should only be substantiated when there is "hard" evidence. Everson and colleagues argue that the research Herman relies on for this opinion is neither representative of nor generalizable to current practice. Everson and colleagues also provide data from their own study of 561 professionals, collected using two different data-collection strategies, to demonstrate the effects of study design on reliability estimates of professional judgments. Finally, Everson and colleagues show how satisfactory interrater reliability can be achieved in case decisions, even when professionals rely on "soft" evidence as the basis of their judgments. Thus, the article by Everson and colleagues challenges the premise that forensic sexual abuse decisions made in the absence of external, corroborative evidence are fundamentally unreliable and unethical. They conclude that Herman's assertions do not represent settled science.

In their article "Mental Health Professionals in Children's Advocacy Centers: Is There Role Conflict?", Cross, Fine, Jones, and Walsh respond to Connell's assertion in Chapter 17 that there is role conflict for the mental health professional who works at or consults with CACs. They also address comparable concerns raised by Melton and Kimbrough-Melton (2006), cited by Connell. Cross and colleagues (this issue), who point out that there were more than 700 Children's Advocacy Centers in the United States at the time they wrote their article. There are standards set by the National Children's Alliance, the membership organization of CACs, which apply to all certified centers. These standards clearly differentiate roles at CACs so as not to create role conflict. Cross and colleagues argue that coordination of the responses of criminal justice, mental health, and other professionals to child abuse is central to CACs mission to promote the *best interests of child victims*. Thus, their article focuses on the interests of children rather than the interest of mental health professionals, which is the primary focus of Connell's Chapter 17. Cross and colleagues assess the risk of conflict of interest by exploring specific mechanisms of and limits to interagency coordination in different CACs. The paper argues that, with best practice, CACs can effectively address both criminal justice and mental health objectives while facilitating sufficient professional autonomy to minimize or eliminate conflict of interest.

Olafson is the author of the article "A Call for Field-Relevant Research About Child Forensic Interviewing for Child Protection." She begins by reminding the reader of the varied and detrimental impacts of child sexual abuse. As the authors did at the beginning of this introduction, Olafson makes the important observation that Kuehnle and Connell's book pays a great deal of attention to the possibility of false positives (false conclusions sexual abuse has occurred) but virtually ignores the far greater problem of false negatives (false conclusions *no* sexual abuse has occurred). Acknowledging the importance to the field and the utility of the NICHD protocol, Olafson points out that this protocol is most useful with children who are in "active disclosure," that is, children who have already provided an account of their sexual abuse to someone, whether a parent or a professional. Olafson therefore calls on the field to develop additional interview methods for children who are reluctant to talk, children who have recanted, very young children, and children with developmental disorders. She notes the emerging body of research supporting extended assessments as a promising development (Faller, Cordisco-Steele, & Nelson-Gardell, 2010; Hershkowitz & Terner, 2007; LaRooy, Lamb et al., 2009).

Finally, Olafson rightly points out that sexual abuse allegations that are evaluated in the context of custody disputes arouse more skepticism and may be given little weight but that very little research has been funded in recent years to learn more about these allegations (Faller & DeVoe, 1995; Thoennes & Tjaden, 1990; Trocme & Bala, 2005). The hypothetical case of Emma, described earlier in this article, is on the verge of being labeled an allegation in a custody dispute, even though Emma's initial spontaneous disclosure was to a therapist agreed upon by both parents when she was exhibiting symptoms they thought were related to their marital discord. This can easily lead to the alleged abuser (in this example the father) receiving custody of Emma in a contested child custody dispute with the mother due to the mother being labeled as the person who programmed the child to make a false allegation and alienated her child against the father.

A TIPPING POINT?

An emphasis on specificity has long dominated the field of forensic assessment of child sexual abuse (Everson, 2010, 2012). Earlier, the authors of this article speculated that when such domination occurs, a tipping point will eventually force a realignment of perspectives. As we have argued, much of the Kuehnle and Connell edited volume presents a strong emphasis on specificity. The question arises whether the Kuehnle and Connell book represents such a tipping point. Or, must we wait for another?

REFERENCES

Adams, J., Harper, K., Knudson, S., & Revilla, J. (1994). Examination findings in legally confirmed child sexual abuse: It's normal to be normal. *Pediatrics, 94,* 310–317.

Bridges, A., Faust, D., & Ahern, D. (2009). Methods for the identification of sexually abused children. In K. Kuehnle & M. Connell (Eds.), *The evaluation of child sexual abuse allegations: A comprehensive guide to assessment and testimony* (pp. 21–47). Hoboken, NJ: John Wiley & Sons.

Brillesljiper-Kater, S., Friedrich, W., & Corwin, D. (2004). Sexual knowledge and emotional reaction as indicators of sexual abuse in young children: Theory and research challenges. *Child Abuse & Neglect, 28,* 1007–1017.

Brown, D., & Lamb, M. (2009). Forensic interviews with children: A two-way street: Supporting interviewers in adhering to best practice recommendations and enhancing children's capabilities in forensic interviews. In K. Kuehnle & M. Connell (Eds.), *The evaluation of child sexual abuse allegations: A comprehensive guide to assessment* (pp. 299–326). New York: John Wiley & Sons.

Buck, J. A., & Warren, A. R. (2009). Jurors and professionals in the legal system: What they know and what they should know about interviewing child witnesses. In K. Kuehnle, & M. Connell (Eds.), *The evaluation of child sexual abuse allegations: A comprehensive guide to assessment and testimony* (pp. 501–530). Hoboken, NJ: John Wiley & Sons.

Cederborg, A., Lamb, M., & Laurell, O. (2007). Delay of disclosure, minimization, and denial of abuse when the evidence is unambiguous: A multivictim case. In M. Pipe, M. Lamb, Y. Orbach, & A. Cederborg (Eds.), *Disclosing abuse: Delays, denials, retractions, and incomplete accounts* (pp. 159–173). Mahwah, NJ: Laurence Earlbaum.

Clark, C. (2009). Professional roles: A key to accuracy and effectiveness. In K. Kuehnle & M. Connell (Eds.), *The evaluation of child sexual abuse allegations: a comprehensive guide to assessment* (pp. 69–80). Hoboken, NJ: Wiley.

Connell, M. (2009a). The child advocacy center model. In K. Kuehnle & M. Connell (Eds.), *The evaluation of child sexual abuse allegations: A comprehensive guide to assessment and testimony* (pp. 423–450). Hoboken, NJ: John Wiley & Sons.

Connell, M. (2009b). The extended forensic evaluation. In K. Kuehnle & M. Connell (Eds.), *The evaluation of child sexual abuse allegations: A comprehensive guide to assessment and testimony* (pp. 451–490). Hoboken, NJ: John Wiley & Sons.

Everson, M. D. (2010). *Contemporary forensic child interviewing: Evolving consensus and innovation over 25 years.* Presentation at When Words Matter Annual Conference, Savannah, GA.

Everson, M. D. (2012, January). *Child forensic interviewing at age 30: Virtuous to a fault.* Presentation at the San Diego International Conference on Child and Family Maltreatment, San Diego, CA.

Everson, M. D., & Sandoval, J. M. (2011). Forensic child sexual abuse evaluations: Assessing subjectivity and bias in professional judgments. *Child Abuse and Neglect, 35*(4), 287–297.

Faller, K. C., Cordisco-Steele, L., & Nelson-Gardell, D. (2010). Allegations of sexual abuse of a child: What to do when a single forensic interview isn't enough. *Journal of Child Sexual Abuse, 19*, 572–589.

Faller, K. C. & DeVoe, E. (1995). Allegations of sexual abuse in divorce. *Journal of Child Sexual Abuse, 4*(4), 1–25.

Faust, D., Bridges, A., & Ahern, D. (2009a). Methods for the identification of sexually abused children: Issues and needed features for abuse indicators. In K. Kuehnle & M. Connell (Eds.), *The evaluation of child sexual abuse allegations: A comprehensive guide to assessment and testimony* (pp. 3–19). Hoboken, NJ: John Wiley & Sons.

Faust, D., Bridges, A., & Ahern, D. (2009b). Methods for the identification of sexually abused children: Suggestions for clinical work and research. In K. Kuehnle & M. Connell (Eds.), *The evaluation of child sexual abuse allegations: A comprehensive guide to assessment and testimony* (pp. 49–66). Hoboken, NJ: John Wiley & Sons.

Friedrich, W. (1993). Sexual victimization and sexual behavior in children: A review of recent literature. *Child Abuse and Neglect, 17*(1), 59–66.

Friedrich, W. (1999). *Child sexual behavior inventory*. Odessa, FL: Psychological Assessment Resources.

Friedrich, W. N. (2002). *Psychological assessment of sexually abused children and their families*. Thousand Oaks, CA: Sage.

Friedrich, W. N., Fisher, J., Dittner, C., Acton, R., Berliner, L., Butler, J., et al. (2001). Child sexual behavior inventory: Normative, psychiatric and sexual abuse comparisons. *Child Maltreatment, 6*, 37–49.

Greenshoot, A., & Tsethlikai, M. (2009). Repressed and recovered memory during childhood and adolescence. In K. Kuehnle & M. Connell (Eds.), *The evaluation of child sexual abuse allegations: A comprehensive guide to assessment* (203–246). Hoboken, NJ: Wiley.

Harris, L., Goodman, G., Augusti, E. M., Chae, Y., & Alley, D. (2009). Children's resistance to suggestion. In K. Kuehnle & M. Connell (Eds.), *The evaluation of child sexual abuse allegations: A comprehensive guide to assessment* (pp. 181–202). Hoboken, NJ: John Wiley & Sons.

Herman, S. (2009). Forensic child sexual abuse evaluations: Accuracy, ethics, and admissibility. In K. Kuehnle & M. Connell (Eds.), *The evaluation of child sexual abuse allegations: A comprehensive guide to assessment* (pp. 247–266). Hoboken, NJ: Wiley.

Hershkowitz, I., Horowitz, D., & Lamb, M. E. (2005). Trends in children's disclosure of abuse in Israel: A national study. *Child Abuse & Neglect, 29*(11), 1203–1214.

Hershkowitz, I., Orbach, Y., Lamb, M., Sternberg, K., Pipe, M., & Horowitz, D. (2006). Dynamics of forensic interviews with suspected abuse victims who do not disclose. *Child Abuse & Neglect, 30*(7), 753–769.

Hershkowitz, I., & Terner, A. (2007). The effects of repeated interviewing on children's forensic statements of sexual abuse. *Applied Cognitive Psychology, 31*, 1131–1143.

Klemfuss, & Ceci, S. (2009). Normative memory development and the child witness. In K. Kuehnle & M. Connell (Eds.), *The evaluation of child sexual abuse allegations: A comprehensive guide to assessment* (pp. 153–180). Hoboken, NJ: Wiley.

Koocher, G. (2009). Ethical issues in child sexual abuse evaluation. In K. Kuehnle & M. Connell (Eds.), *The evaluation of child sexual abuse allegations: A comprehensive guide to assessment* (pp. 81–100). Hoboken, NJ: Wiley.

Kuehnle, K., & Connell, M. (2009). *The evaluation of child sexual abuse allegations: A comprehensive guide to assessment.* Hoboken, NJ: Wiley.

Kuehnle, K., & Connell, M. (2010). Child sexual abuse suspicions: Treatment considerations during investigation. *Journal of Child Sexual Abuse, 19*, 554–571.

La Rooy, D., Lamb, M., Pipe, M. E. (2009). Repeated interviews: A recritical evaluation of risks and benefits. In K. Kuehnle & M. Connell (Eds.), *The evaluation of child sexual abuse allegations: A comprehensive guide to assessment* (pp. 327–364). Hoboken, NJ: John Wiley & Sons.

Lamb, M. E., Hershkowitz, I., Orbach, Y., & Esplin, P. W. (2008). *Tell me what happened. Structured investigative interviews of child victims and witnesses.* West Sussex, England: Wiley-Blackwell.

Lamb, M., Orbach, Y., Hershkowitz, I., Esplin, P., & Horowitz, D. (2007). A structured forensic interview protocol improves the quality and informativeness of investigative interviews with children: A review of research using the NICHD investigative interview protocol. *Child Abuse & Neglect, 31*, 1201–1231.

London, K., Bruck, M., Ceci, S., & Shuman, D. (2005). Disclosure of child sexual abuse: What does the research tell us about how children tell? *Psychology, Public Policy, and the Law, 11*, 194–226.

Malloy, L., & Quas, J. (2009). Children's suggestibility: Areas of consensus and controversy. In K. Kuehnle & M. Connell (Eds.), *The evaluation of child sexual abuse allegations: A comprehensive guide to assessment* (pp. 267–298). Hoboken, NJ: John Wiley & Sons.

Melton, G. B. & Kimbrough-Melton, R. J. (2006). Integrating assessment, treatment and jusice: Pipe dream or possibility. In S. N. Sparta & G.P. Koocher (Eds.), *Forensic mental health assessment of children and adolescents* (pp. 30–45). New York: Oxford University Press.

Myers, J. E. B. (2009). Improving forensic interviewing: The legacy of the McMartin Pre-school case. In K. Kuehnle & M. Connell (Eds.), *The evaluation of child sexual abuse allegations: A comprehensive guide to assessment* (pp. xix–xxv). Hoboken, NJ: John Wiley & Sons.

Pipe, M., Lamb, M. E., Orbach, Y., Sternberg, K. J., Stewart, H. L., & Esplin, P. W. (2007). Factors associated with nondisclosure of suspected abuse during forensic interviews. In M. Pipe, M. Lamb, Y. Orbach, & A. Cederborg (Eds.), *Child sexual abuse: Disclosure, delay, and denial* (pp. 77–96). Mahwah, NJ: Lawrence Erlbaum.

Pipe, M. E., & Salmon, K. (2009). Dolls, drawing, body diagrams, and others props: Role of props in investigative interviews. In K. Kuehnle & M. Connell (Eds.), *The evaluation of child sexual abuse allegations: A comprehensive guide to assessment* (pp. 365–396). Hoboken, NJ: John Wiley & Sons.

Poole, D., & Wolfe, M. (2009). Child development: Normative sexual and nonsexual behaviors that may be confused with symptoms of sexual abuse. In K. Kuehnle & M. Connell (Eds.), *The evaluation of child sexual abuse allegations:*

A comprehensive guide to assessment (pp. 101–128). Hoboken, NJ: John Wiley & Sons.

Sas, L., & Cunningham, A. (1995). *Tipping the balance to tell the secret: The Public discovery of child sexual abuse*. London, Ontario, Canada: London Court Clinic.

Shuman, D. W., & Austin, B. G. (2009). The return of the ultimate issue: Talking to the court in child sexual abuse cases. In K. Kuehnle, M. Connell, K. Kuehnle, M. Connell (Eds.), *The evaluation of child sexual abuse allegations: A comprehensive guide to assessment and testimony* (pp. 491–499). Hoboken, NJ: John Wiley & Sons.

Thoennes, N., & Tjaden, P. (1990). The extent, nature, and validity of sexual abuse allegations in custody/visitation disputes. *Child Abuse & Neglect, 14,* 151–63.

Trocme, N., & Bala, N. (2005). False allegations of abuse and neglect when parents separate. *Child Abuse & Neglect, 29,* 1333–1345.

AUTHOR NOTES

Kathleen Coulborn Faller, PhD, ACSW, DCSW, is Marion Elizabeth Blue Professor of Children and Families in the School of Social Work at the University of Michigan and Director of the Family Assessment Clinic, a program at the University of Michigan School of Social Work that involves collaboration with the Law School and the Medical School. She is Principal Investigator on Training Program on Recruitment and Retention of Child Welfare Workers and Principal Investigator of the University of Michigan site of National Child Welfare Workforce Institute.

Mark D. Everson, PhD, is Professor of Psychiatry and Director of the Program on Childhood Trauma and Maltreatment at the University of North Carolina at Chapel Hill.

DIAGNOSTIC UTILITY OF THE ALLEGED CHILD VICTIM'S DISCLOSURE STATEMENT AND BEHAVIOR SYMPTOMS

Interviewing Children Versus Tossing Coins: Accurately Assessing the Diagnosticity of Children's Disclosures of Abuse

THOMAS D. LYON, ELIZABETH C. AHERN,
and NICHOLAS SCURICH
University of Southern California, Los Angeles, California, USA

We describe a Bayesian approach to evaluating children's abuse disclosures and review research demonstrating that children's disclosure of genital touch can be highly probative of sexual abuse, with the probative value depending on disclosure spontaneity and children's age. We discuss how some commentators understate the probative value of children's disclosures by: confusing the probability of abuse given disclosure with the probability of disclosure given abuse, assuming that children formally questioned about sexual abuse have a low prior probability of sexual abuse, misstating the probative value of abuse disclosure, and confusing the distinction between disclosure and nondisclosure with the distinction between true and false disclosures. We review interviewing methods that increase the probative value of disclosures, including interview instructions, narrative practice, noncontingent reinforcement, and questions about perpetrator/caregiver statements and children's reactions to the alleged abuse.

Because the child victim tends to be the only eyewitness to sexual abuse (other than the perpetrator), the child's report is an extremely important piece of evidence in any abuse case. Researchers have identified a number of ways in which child interviewing can be improved, both by increasing the number of true details in reports of children who have been abused and by decreasing the likelihood that children who have not been abused make false reports. We will argue that children's disclosures of abuse can be highly probative of abuse, particularly when they are elicited using techniques supported by research.

Kuehnle and Connell (2009) brought together a diverse group of scholars with widely varying views regarding the potential to distinguish between true and false suspicions of child sexual abuse. The first three chapters, authored by David Faust and colleagues, took a Bayesian approach to understanding the process by which evaluators attempt to determine if abuse has occurred (Bridges, Faust, & Ahern, 2009; Faust, Bridges, & Ahern, 2009a, 2009b). They painted a pessimistic picture regarding the ability of research on abused and nonabused children to increase the diagnostic accuracy of sexual abuse assessments. We agree that the Bayesian approach is an excellent framework for understanding the difficulties of evaluating abuse allegations. However, we will argue that Faust and colleagues' examples may lead one to underestimate the value of disclosures of abuse.

Chapters by Brown and Lamb (2009) and Herman (2009) discussed the National Institutes of Child Health and Human Development (NICHD) protocol for interviewing children about abuse. Brown and Lamb (2009) reviewed evidence that the NICHD protocol increases the quantity and quality of information that children questioned about abuse provide. We agree and will elaborate on interviewing methods that can increase the diagnosticity of disclosures. Herman (2009) argued that the NICHD protocol does a poor job of distinguishing between true and false allegations of abuse. We believe that Herman understated the probative evidentiary value of a disclosure of abuse and the advantages of the NICHD protocol.

First, we will present a primer on Bayesian thinking about probabilities. This is intended to introduce the subject to novice readers. Second, we will critique Faust and colleagues' discussion of the probative value of sexual abuse indicators. We will explain how they fell prey to the inverse fallacy in their argument about the limited probative value of indicators. We will also argue that they underestimated the likelihood that children seen for sexual abuse assessment have been abused because of the likelihood that assessment is triggered by disclosure. Third, we will discuss the probative value of children's disclosures of genital touch and argue that such disclosures often have very high probative value, taking into account the child's age and the type of questions asked in assessing disclosure. Fourth, we will discuss innovations in interviewing that increase probative value, including interview instructions and open-ended narrative practice. Fifth, we will take issue with Herman's pessimistic conclusions about the probative value of children's disclosures.

THE BAYESIAN APPROACH: UNDERSTANDING HOW TO ASSESS EVIDENCE OF ABUSE

Before we discuss other authors' treatment of the diagnosticity of disclosures, it is important to describe the Bayesian approach (Bolstad, 2007). A mainstay of probability theory is Bayes's theorem. Bayes's theorem formally prescribes the extent to which one ought to update one's belief in a given proposition in light of receiving new information. According to the theorem, one updates one's belief by multiplying the *prior probability* of the proposition by the value of the new information (Lyon & Koehler, 1996). Let's imagine that we are attempting to determine the probability that a child was abused and that the new information is "this child disclosed sexual abuse in a forensic interview." The prior probability is the probability that the child was abused based on all we knew about the child before considering the child's disclosure.

If the child was randomly selected from the population to be questioned about sexual abuse, the prior probability would be equal to the base rate of abuse among children in the population. Faust and colleagues (2009a, 2009b), for example, assumed an abuse base rate of 5%. We will return to the issue of base rates later, but for now it is important to understand that we would use the base rate as the prior probability if we had no reason to suspect abuse before we learned that the child disclosed abuse in an interview.

Bayes's theorem is easiest to understand if one speaks in terms of odds rather than percentages. For example, if the likelihood of abuse is 50%, this is even odds; the likelihood the child was abused (50%) is equal to the likelihood that the child was not abused (50%). Odds can be expressed as a ratio; even odds would be 1:1. It is not very difficult to convert percentages to odds ratios. The percentage likelihood is the first value in the ratio and 100 minus the percentage likelihood is the second value in the odds ratio. Hence, if the likelihood of abuse is 50%, 50 is the first value in the odds ratio. The second value is 100 minus 50, or 50. So for a 50% likelihood, the odds ratio is 50:50, which simplifies to 1:1. If one assumes a base rate of 5%, then the odds would be 5:(100–5) or 5:95, which simplifies to 1:19.[1]

The value of the new information (which can be called the probative value or the diagnosticity) is typically quantified as a *likelihood ratio*. The likelihood ratio is the ratio of the true positive rate and the false positive rate. The true positive rate is the likelihood that children disclose abuse when they *have* been abused. The false positive rate is the likelihood that children disclose abuse when they have *not* been abused. In other words, the likelihood ratio will be the proportion of abused children who disclose abuse divided by the proportion of nonabused children who disclose abuse. For example, assume that 40% of abused children disclose abuse, whereas 2% of nonabused children falsely claim abuse. The likelihood ratio for disclosure is the proportion of abused children who disclose abuse (40%) divided by the proportion of nonabused children who disclose abuse (2%), or 20.

The likelihood ratio indicates how much the odds of abuse are increased by the new information (the disclosure). A likelihood ratio of 20 means that the evidence increases the odds of abuse 20 times. Hence, in order to calculate the likelihood that a child who discloses abuse was in fact abused, we multiply the prior odds by the likelihood ratio. Thus, if the prior odds of abuse are 1:19 and the likelihood ratio is 20, the likelihood of abuse is 20:19, which is slightly higher than 1:1 odds.

Imagine that a child is randomly selected from a group of children, only 5% of whom were abused. This would mean that the prior probability of abuse, before we interview the child, would be equal to the base rate of abuse: only 5%, or 1:19 odds. Then imagine that the child is interviewed about abuse, and discloses abuse, and the likelihood ratio of a disclosure is 20. We would then conclude that the odds that the child really was abused was 20:19, or only slightly better than 1:1. In percentage terms, it would be 51%.[2]

Commentators sometimes describe likelihood ratios as being strong or weak evidence. For example, Wood (1996) notes that a likelihood ratio of 3 is considered weak, 5 weak to moderate, 7 moderate, 14 moderate-to-strong, and 20 strong. But even strong evidence may not be convincing if the prior odds of abuse are very low (Faust et al., 2009a, 2009b; Myers, 2005; Poole & Wolfe, 2009). Indeed, the example we just discussed is an illustration of this problem. We assumed that disclosure has a likelihood ratio of 20, which makes disclosure strong evidence. But because the prior odds of abuse were only 1:19, disclosure makes it only slightly more probable than not that the child was abused.

On the other hand, if one starts with high prior odds, even a likelihood ratio that is considered weak can convince one that abuse occurred. It is unusual for children to be plucked at random from the population and given a forensic interview for abuse. To the extent that evidence of abuse exists before the child is interviewed, then the prior probability of abuse is likely to be much higher than the base rate. For example, if the prior odds are 1:1, then a likelihood ratio of three increases the odds to 3:1 or 75%. In other words, one might be on the fence before the disclosure but firmly convinced after the disclosure.

There are two other important points to make about the likelihood ratio. The reader will recall that we assumed 40% of abused children disclose abuse (the true positive rate) and 2% of nonabused children disclose abuse (the false positive rate). Forty percent is a minority of abused children. However, 2% is a very small number, so even if most abused children deny abuse, disclosure can be strong evidence of abuse. Similarly, the fact that evidence is common or rare among abused children tells us very little about the diagnosticity of that evidence. Imagine that 60% of abused children experience nightmares. This may mean nothing at all if 60% of nonabused children experience nightmares. On the other hand, imagine that 1% of abused children suffer from gonorrhea. This may be very strong evidence of abuse if the percentage of nonabused children who suffer from gonorrhea is much less than 1%. Hence, the likelihood ratio teaches us that we cannot assess the diagnosticity of any piece of evidence without knowing both the true positive rate *and* the false positive rate (Lyon & Koehler, 1996).

A second point is that it is very important not to confuse the different terms. The true positive rate and the false positive rate are quite different. Knowing the true positive rate does not tell us what the false positive rate is. Novices will sometimes assume that the true and false positive rates must sum to one, which is incorrect. They are calculated based on different groups of children: the true positive rate is calculated based on abused children, and the false positive rate is based on nonabused children.

It is also easy to confuse the true positive rate with the probability of abuse given disclosure. The true positive rate is the probability of *disclosure given abuse*. The reader should notice that this sounds similar to the probability of *abuse given disclosure*. Confusion between these two probabilities has been given different names: the inverse fallacy (Kaye & Koehler, 1991), transposing the conditional (Evett, 1995), and the prosecutor's fallacy (Thompson & Schumann, 1987). We will use the term inverse fallacy.

COIN TOSSES VERSUS TESTS THAT ARE 75 % ACCURATE

Now we are ready to consider the arguments made by Faust and his colleagues (Bridges et al., 2009; Faust et al., 2009 a, 2009b). They purported to show that a test that is 75% accurate may nevertheless be worse than a coin toss in distinguishing between true and false allegations of abuse. If their proposition is true, it would indeed undermine one's confidence in assessing child sexual abuse claims. However, the "75% accurate" argument suffers from two principal problems that may mislead the novice reader. First, the "75% accurate" test is actually only weakly probative, with a likelihood ratio of three. Understanding how Faust and colleagues define "accurate" will make this clear. Second, the "75% accurate" test is in fact stronger evidence than a coin toss. Because of looseness in the meaning of the term "accurate," Faust and colleagues fell prey to the inverse fallacy.

Faust et al. (2009a) wrote, "Assume there is an evaluative method or test with a 75% accuracy rate in separating [abused children from non-abused children]. Although 75% is far from perfect, it might well seem that the test has much to offer and could help us" (p. 10). Seventy-five percent certainly sounds like a good test. The reader might assume that if a test is 75% accurate, this means that if the test says the child is abused, it is 75% likely to be correct. Surely, if it is correct 75% of the time, then it could be usable as a means of distinguishing abused children from nonabused children.

However, Faust and colleagues used the term "accuracy" in a specific and somewhat idiosyncratic way. They described a test that has a 75% true positive rate *and* a 75% true *negative* rate. So, if the child was abused, the evidence would be present 75% of the time (the true positive rate). If the child was not abused, the evidence would be absent 75% of the time (the true negative rate). In order to assess the value of the "75% accurate" test, one needs to know the likelihood ratio. The numerator of the likelihood ratio is the true positive rate, and the denominator is the false positive rate. The true positive rate of the "75% accurate test" is 75%. The false positive rate can easily be calculated using the true negative rate. The false positive rate of the "75% accurate" test is 25%.[3] This means that the "75% accurate" test has a likelihood ratio of only three.

Translating the "75% accurate" test into a likelihood ratio gives us a better picture of how useful the test is. The likelihood ratio of three is considered weak evidence, and a false positive rate of 25% is quite high. For example, if the evidence in question was a disclosure of abuse, then a false positive rate of 25% would mean that the questioning method elicited false claims of abuse from 25% of nonabused children. Indeed, a false positive rate of 25% ensures that the evidence will be weak; the highest possible likelihood ratio is four because the true positive rate cannot be greater than 100%.

Furthermore, translating the "75% accurate" test into a likelihood ratio emphasizes the need to consider the prior odds of abuse. Faust and colleagues made the correct point that if one starts with a low probability of abuse and finds weak evidence of abuse (the "75% accurate" test), the likelihood of abuse will remain low. They discussed two different cases, either assuming a prior probability of abuse of 17% (equal to a prior odds of 1:5) or 50% (prior odds of 1:1). In the case in which the prior probability of abuse is 17%, a positive result on the "75% accurate" test would increase the odds of abuse by three, from 1:5 to 3:5, or 38%. If the prior probability is 50%, then a positive test result would increase the odds of abuse by three, from 1:1 to 3:1, or 75%.

With respect to the 38% figure, Faust and colleagues (2009a) concluded, "[W]e will be wrong far more often than we are correct: our accuracy rate will only be 38%, or worse than a coin toss, an outcome that is hardly satisfactory" (p. 12). This is an example of the inverse fallacy. The problem lies in the ambiguity of the term "accuracy rate." The authors start with the assumption that the "accuracy rate" of a coin toss is 50%. However, by comparing coin tosses to the 38% "accuracy rate," the authors confused the probability of evidence given abuse (50%, using a coin toss) to the probability of abuse given evidence (38%).

To demonstrate the inverse fallacy, consider how a coin toss can be considered both 50% accurate (likelihood of evidence given abuse) and less than 50% accurate (likelihood of abuse given evidence). Imagine that you take a group of 100 children, 10 of whom have been abused, and you toss a coin to determine who is abused and who is not abused: heads abused, tails nonabused. If you take any child who has been abused and toss a coin, the likelihood that you will call the child abused is 50%. Hence, the coin appears to be 50% "accurate." But now consider the entire group of children. By tossing coins, you will randomly select 50 of the 100 children "as abused." The proportion of the 50 children who really will have been abused will be the same as the original group: 10%. Therefore, the coin toss will only be correct 10% of the time. Hence, the probability of abuse given heads is 10%, but the probability of heads given abuse is 50%. The two probabilities are quite different and should not be confused.

By committing the inverse fallacy, Faust and colleagues were able to dismiss the use of relevant evidence. The truth of the matter is that evidence with a likelihood ratio of three increases the odds of abuse by three times. A coin toss does not affect the odds of abuse (and we do not recommend using it!). If the prior probability is low, it will remain low in the face of this weak evidence. But if the prior probability is close to 50% (or 1:1) odds, this evidence can make the difference. In sum, Faust and colleagues' argument purported to show that a test can be 75% accurate and yet worse than a coin flip. Their "75% accurate" test is only weakly diagnostic (likelihood ratio of three) and nevertheless clearly better than a coin toss.

UNREALISTIC ASSUMPTIONS ABOUT THE LIKELIHOOD OF ABUSE AMONG CHILDREN SEEN FOR EVALUATION

Faust and colleagues rightly speculated that children are typically evaluated for sexual abuse because "someone suspects abuse" (Bridges, Faust, & Ahern, 2009, p. 25). The relevance of the suspicion, however, is very important. In their hypothetical example, Faust and colleagues discussed the use of a "screening method with robust validity" (Faust, Bridges, & Ahern, 2009a, p. 11) and assumed the following numbers:

> For purposes of this example, assume that the base rate for child sexual abuse in the catchment area for Clinic 1 is 5%. Thus, there are 19 non-abused children for every sexually abused child. Assume that all children

known to display explicit sexual behavior, such as imitating sexual relations with dolls, are referred for sexual abuse evaluations. Assume further that explicit sexual behavior occurs in about 20% of sexually abused children and 5% of non-abused children (figures that roughly align with research estimates. . .). (p. 11)

The evidence—sexual play with dolls—has a likelihood ratio of 4 (true positive rate = 20%; false positive rate = 5%), which would be considered "weak" evidence. If one starts with a base rate of 5% (or 1:19 odds), multiplying this by a likelihood ratio of 4 leaves us with 4:19 or approximately 1:5 odds of abuse. This is only 17%. The 17% figure is the one that the authors use, in conjunction with the "75% accurate" test, to argue that coin tosses are better than abuse evaluations.

We will not challenge the assumption that 5% is a reasonable base rate for the population. As others in this special issue emphasize, the prevalence of abuse among children is substantially higher than 5%, particularly among girls (Everson & Faller, this issue). However, we are not sure that the prevalence rate is the correct base rate. The prevalence rate is the percentage of children who are abused at any time during childhood, but many children are questioned long before their childhood ends, and therefore the likelihood they will have been abused will be lower.

What we find questionable about the hypothetical is that it assumes communities screen for sexual abuse by giving children at large anatomically correct dolls with which to play. It is hard to imagine that anyone would ever undertake such an approach. First, we are not aware of any screening of children at large for sexual abuse. Second, if we did conduct population screening, it is unlikely that we would have children play with anatomical dolls. A fairly broad consensus has emerged that observation of doll play is not a valid means of evaluating children for sexual abuse. Rather, supporters of the use of dolls advocate their use as a demonstration aid for children who are disclosing abuse (Pipe & Salmon, 2009).

The fact is that disclosure is a common, if not the most common, reason children are evaluated for sexual abuse. For example, Heger, Ticson, Valsquez, and Bernier (2002) examined the records of 2,400 children referred for evaluation of sexual abuse and found that 70% of the children had previously disclosed abuse.

THE DIAGNOSTICITY OF THE DISCLOSURE OF GENITAL TOUCH

It is therefore most relevant to consider the diagnosticity of the disclosure of abuse in determining the likelihood that professional evaluations of abuse allegations are correct. The evidence suggests that children's spontaneous reports of genital touching are strong evidence that touching has occurred but that as the questions become more direct and potentially leading, and as younger children are questioned, the diagnosticity of a report of genital touch decreases.

For example, an oft-cited study by Saywitz, Goodman, Nicholas, and Moan (1991) examined 72 five- and seven-year-olds girls' memories of a pediatric examination. For half of the girls, the examination included genital touch, and for the other half, the examiner substituted an examination for scoliosis. When asked free recall questions about the event one month afterward, 22% of the girls who had been touched mentioned vaginal touch, and none of the girls who had not been touched did so. When asked a direct question about genital touch with the aid of an anatomically correct doll ("Did that doctor touch you there?" while pointing to the doll's vagina, p. 684), 86% of the girls who had been touched acknowledged genital touch and 3% of the girls who had not been touched falsely claimed that they had. The results suggest that a spontaneous report of genital touch (in response to a very general question about one's interactions with a person) is very strong evidence. We might say that the likelihood ratio is infinitely large, although it would be safer to say that in this study recall of genital touch provided conclusive proof that touching occurred. Even a simple "yes" response to a direct question with an anatomically correct doll constituted strong evidence of genital touch (86/3, or a likelihood ratio of 29).

Steward and colleagues (1996) conducted a similar study in which children were either touched or not touched during a physical exam. However, they included children from three to six years of age, used either anatomically detailed dolls or anatomical body diagrams, and interviewed the children one day, one month, and six months after the exam. Direct questions about genital touch asked with the assistance of a doll or drawing elicited relatively weak evidence of touching; the likelihood ratios ranged from five to nine. True positive rates ranged from 73% to 86%, whereas false positive rates ranged from 8% to 12%. In contrast, when children were asked, "Did the doctor touch you?" and then, if they answered yes, were asked, "Where were you touched?" there were no false reports of genital touch in the verbal-only interviews at any of the time periods, whereas the true positive rates ranged from 18% to 33%. Disclosure of genital touching without the use of dolls or drawings constituted conclusive evidence of touch. Three-year-olds performed worse than six-year-olds.

Indeed, as younger children are tested, the false positive rates increase, making direct questions with dolls increasingly risky. Bruck and colleagues (Bruck, Ceci, Francouer, & Renick, 1995, Bruck, Ceci, & Francouer, 2000) questioned preschool children immediately after a pediatric examination and included direct questions with the aid of an anatomically detailed doll. Some of the questions were highly suggestive, but we will only consider the questions about genital touch most analogous to those asked by Saywitz and colleagues (1991) and Steward and colleagues (1996): yes–no questions that asked whether the doctor touched the child's genitalia. Although Bruck and colleagues did not find significant age differences, their sample sizes were small and the percentages suggested improvement with age. The three-year-olds (mean age 2 years 11 months) performed close to chance, such that the likelihood ratio was not greater than one. Specifically, children exhibited a 50% true positive rate and a 42% false positive rate. The four-year-olds (mean age 4 years 1 month) exhibited a 45% true positive rate and a 14% false positive rate, which suggests a likelihood ratio of 3, or weak evidence of touching.

Critics of the Saywitz and colleagues (1991) and Steward and colleagues (1996) studies have pointed out that they did not contain a number of other suggestive elements that may occur when children are questioned about abuse, particularly when the questioner strongly suspects that abuse has occurred (Bruck & Ceci, 1996, 1999). Critics also focus on the false positive rate for anal touch, which is often inexplicably quite a lot higher (Bruck & Ceci, 1996). Indeed, because of the increased false alarm rate with the use of anatomical dolls or drawings, we have cautioned against their use (Lyon, Lamb, & Myers, 2009). Hence, this discussion is not intended as a defense of the use of dolls but rather illustrates the fact that even methods criticized as unduly suggestive will often elicit reports that increase the likelihood that genital touching occurred, particularly with children older than preschool age.

To our knowledge, researchers have not asked about genital touch when using more suggestive methods. They have, however, asked questions that would strongly intimate that genital touching may have occurred. For example, Bruck & Ceci (2004) summarize one study as finding a 68% false positive rate for "misleading questions with abuse themes (e.g., 'He took your clothes off, didn't he?')" when the questions are asked in a high-pressure interview (p. 231, citing Finnila, Mahlberga, Santtilaa, & Niemib, 2003).

Finnila and colleagues (2003) tested four- and eight-year-old children who were either the most suggestible or least suggestible in their age groups. Children participated in a 10-minute interaction with an adult male and were questioned one week later. In the "low pressure" group, children were asked questions such as, "He took your clothes off, didn't he?" In the "high pressure" group, children were first told, "I have already spoken to the big kids and they told me that he did some bad things that he shouldn't have done. Now I would like to know if you also have such a good memory and can help me, because I really need your help to find out what happened." For each question, the interviewer first told the child what other children had reported (e.g., "The other kids told me that he took their clothes off. He took your clothes off too, didn't he?" If the child said "yes" or "maybe," the interviewer "praised the child's memory." If the child said "no," the interviewer implied that the child's answer might be wrong, repeated what "the other kids" had said, and re-asked the question. Again, if the child now said "yes" or "maybe," the interviewer praised the child's memory; p. 42).

Although Bruck and Ceci (2004) report a 68% false positive rate for misleading questions generally, citing the "clothes off" question as an example, Finnila and colleagues (2003) report specific percentages for the "clothes off" question. In the "high pressure" condition, 9% of children answered "yes" to "He took your clothes off, didn't he?" In the "low pressure" condition 3% did so. The rate in the "high pressure" condition is significantly higher than in the "low pressure" condition, but at the same time, given the pressures inflicted on the child subjects, remarkably low.

We would never advocate the use of the high-pressure tactics, but if they have been used, an important question is whether the child's responses are nondiagnostic. Given a 9% false positive rate, if the high-pressure interview elicited a true positive rate of 60% or more, then a "yes" response would be considered moderately strong evidence. However, because Finnila and colleagues (2003) did not test a condition in which clothes were in fact removed, one cannot assess the diagnosticity of children's "yes" responses to the "clothes off" questions.

Similar to the anatomical dolls research, the questions are likely to elicit higher error rates in younger children. Goodman and Aman (1990) interviewed three- and five-year-old children (some with anatomical dolls) about a ten-minute interaction with a man and asked the "clothes off" question as part of a group of suggestive questions ("He took your clothes off, didn't he?" "He kissed you, didn't he?" and "How many times did he spank you?"). Whereas three-year-olds false alarmed 21% of the time, five-year-olds did so only 2% of the time (p. 1867). Similarly, the authors asked children more directly about genital touch ("Did he touch your private parts?" "Did he keep his clothes on?" and "Show me where he touched you"). Whereas 14% of the three-year-olds' responses "would be likely to raise suspicions of abuse," 5% of the five-year-olds responses were so coded (p. 1865). In contrast, Finnila and colleagues (2003) report no age differences. However, they did find that children's accuracy was related to their performance on a suggestibility scale, and that scale, in turn, was related to age. Hence, by testing the effects of both the suggestibility scale and age in the same model, the effect of age may have been captured (and thus obscured) by the effect of the scale.

In sum, the fact that a child has disclosed genital touch has substantial probative value in concluding that the child was sexually abused. If the child reports abuse in free recall, this is arguably very strong evidence of abuse, and even if the child's disclosure is only in response to more direct questions, this has some probative value. As children mature, their "yes" responses to direct questions increase in probative value.

THE POTENTIAL REDUNDANCY OF DISCLOSURE

When children are referred for evaluation of sexual abuse, they are obviously questioned about abuse. If most referred children are referred because of a disclosure, this means that the evaluation will include both the child's previous statements and any disclosure the child makes during the evaluation. Faust and colleagues (Bridges, Faust, & Ahern, 2009) raised a potential problem with double-counting evidence, one that they called double-dipping. The evaluator should not assume that the child's responses during the evaluation are independent of the child's prior disclosure. As they wrote, "[T]he problem is that once the variable or variables have been used during Phase 1 as a basis for referral, then any positive qualities they might have had for the detection of abuse are neutralized when they are reapplied in Phase 2, with the result often being to reduce judgmental accuracy" (p. 29). Faust and colleagues noted that redundant information adds no incremental validity to the assessment but may lead to overconfidence in the judgment about the occurrence of abuse because of the evaluator's failure to recognize redundancy.

Faust and colleagues applied this reasoning to sexual behavior. Does it also apply to interviewing? In order for the new disclosure to add nothing to the evaluator's judgment, the second disclosure must be truly redundant. However, there are a number of reasons why the evaluation interview will not be redundant, particularly if it relies as much as possible on open-ended questions.

First, the child's initial disclosure is likely to have contained few details. Children's first reports are rarely to the authorities, and nonprofessionals are unlikely to conduct exhaustive forensic interviews when children first disclose. Second, if the child's disclosure was to an interested person (such as a parent involved in a custody dispute with the accused), then there are sure to be doubts about the credibility of that person's report. The disclosure may never have occurred at all, may have been ambiguous and subject to misinterpretation, or may have been elicited through leading questions. Third, even if the recipient of the report was unbiased, the child's report may have been elicited through direct questions, which would reduce the diagnosticity of the disclosure because responses to direct questions tend to be less accurate than free recall. To the extent that the evaluation interview is more open-ended and less leading than the interaction that led to the child's initial disclosure, the diagnosticity of the evaluation interview increases. Some suggestibility research documents that errors in response to suggestive questions may persevere or increase over multiple interviews, but this is far from inevitable; these effects emerge when each interview is itself suggestive and highly leading questions are asked (LaRooy, Lamb, & Pipe, 2009; Goodman & Quas, 2008). A large component of suggestibility is due to errors in the child's responses rather than impairment of the child's memory, which means that nonleading questions will not elicit repeated errors. On the other hand, repeated open-ended interviews are likely to reveal a great deal of new and accurate information (LaRooy et al., 2009). Furthermore, the evaluation interview need not yield any new information to be valuable. The interview is likely to be what Schum and Martin (1982) called *corroboratively redundant*. The redundant report is corroborative of abuse because it reduces worries regarding the validity of the initial disclosure.

INTERVIEWING METHODS FOR INCREASING THE DIAGNOSTICITY OF ABUSE DISCLOSURES

Although the bulk of research on children's suggestibility has emphasized the ways in which children's accuracy can be impaired, a growing number of studies have explored means of increasing the accuracy and completeness of children's reports. These techniques will increase the diagnosticity of disclosures of abuse to the extent that they increase the likelihood that abused children will disclose (true positives) and decrease the likelihood of false disclosures (false positives).

Interviewers who begin with interview instructions can increase the accuracy of children's reports. It is recommended that interviewers (a) teach children that they can say "I don't know" (Cordon, Saetermoe, & Goodman, 2005) because children may be reluctant to respond "I don't know" to yes–no questions (Poole & Lindsay, 2001) or specific wh- questions (e.g., "What color was his hat?") (e.g., Memon & Vartoukian, 1996); (b) teach children that they can say "I don't understand" (Saywitz, Snyder, & Nathanson, 1999; Peters & Nunez, 1999) because children frequently fail to ask for clarification (Carter, Bottoms, & Levine, 1996; Perry, McAuliff, Tan, & Claycomb, 1995; Saywitz, et al., 1999); and (c) teach children that they can correct the interviewer (Saywitz & Moan-Hardie, 1994; Warren, Hulse-Trotter, & Tubbs, 1991). Interviewers are encouraged to not only explain the rules of the interview but also to provide children examples, because an unelaborated instruction (e.g., "It's okay to say I don't know") is unlikely to be effective (Geddie, Fradin, & Beer, 2000; Memon & Vartoukian, 1996; Moston, 1987). Furthermore, interviewers should reinforce giving an answer when one can so that children do not overutilize the "don't know" or "don't understand" responses (Gee, Gregory, & Pipe, 1999; Saywitz & Moan-Hardie, 1994). Eliciting a promise to tell the truth from children has been found to increase honesty without increasing errors (Evans & Lee, 2010, Lyon & Dorado, 2008; Talwar, Lee, Bala, & Lindsay, 2002, 2004), even among maltreated children who have been coached to either falsely deny or falsely claim that events occurred (Lyon, Malloy, Quas, & Talwar, 2008).

Interviewers who elicit abuse details through open-ended questions increase accuracy. As noted, children's free recall reports of genital touch are much more probative than "yes" responses to closed-ended questions.

In general, children's free recall reports are much more accurate than their responses to recognition questions (Dale, Loftus, & Rathbun, 1978; Dent, 1982, 1986; Dent & Stephenson, 1979; Goodman & Aman, 1990; Goodman, Bottoms, Schwartz-Kenney, & Rudy, 1991; Hutcheson, Baxter, Telfer, & Warden, 1995; Oates & Shrimpton, 1991; Ornstein, Gordon & Larus, 1992).

When children are properly questioned, questions tapping free recall can elicit surprisingly large amounts of information. In forensic interviews, children's responses to free recall prompts elicited three to five times more information than responses to more focused prompts (Lamb, Hershkowitz, Orbach, & Esplin, 2008). The key is to provide the child some guidance. Laboratory studies demonstrating very poor recall performance among younger children led some commentators to conclude that direct questions may be necessary in order to elicit abuse details (Lyon, 1999), but the limitation of those studies is that free recall questions did little more than ask "What happened?" "What else happened?" and "Tell me more." In contrast, an interviewer who asks follow-up questions in the form of "You said x; tell me more about x" or "You said x; what happened next?" elicits free recall while providing the child needed scaffolding.

Children are not accustomed to being asked open-ended questions, and they benefit from practice. A useful tool is narrative practice in which the interviewer asks the child about an innocuous event before moving to the allegation. For example, the interviewer asks the child to "Tell me everything that happened" on the child's last birthday, and seeks elaboration through "You said x, what happened next" and "You said x; tell me more about x" questions. In the field, Sternberg and colleagues (1997) found that when interviewers used narrative practice during rapport-building with open-ended rather than closed-ended questions, children provided longer and richer responses to the first substantive question about abuse, and longer responses to free recall questions throughout the interview. Laboratory research has demonstrated that children's responses are also more accurate when narrative practice is provided before the substantive interview (Roberts, Lamb, & Sternberg, 2004).

Narrative practice can profitably be combined with nonsuggestive forms of interviewer encouragement and support. Addressing the child by his or her name and providing noncontingent reinforcement (e.g., "You really help me understand") is related to greater elaboration by the child (Hershkowitz, 2009). Another form of reinforcement is the use of facilitators, also known as back-channel responses, in which the interviewer encourages additional information through simple utterances that communicate that the interviewer is listening without taking the floor (e.g., "uh huh," "okay"; Cautilli, Riley-Tillman, Axelrod, & Hineline, 2005). Laboratory research has also found that interviewer social support, such as smiling often, using warm vocal intonations, and sitting in close proximity helps children resist misleading questions (Davis & Bottoms, 2002).

Reinforcement is noncontingent to the extent that the interviewer does not *selectively reinforce* desired responses. Contingent reinforcement, on the other hand, can be highly leading, particularly when the interviewer overtly praises acquiescence to yes–no questions (Garven, Wood, Malpass, & Shaw, 1998, 2000). Analogously, when examining child interviews regarding a mild transgression, general reassurance about disclosing negative information increased children's true disclosures (Lyon et al. 2008), but reassurance that specifically mentioned the transgression increased false positives (Lyon & Dorado, 2008).

We recommend that interviewers encountering reluctance inform the child that "it is really important that I know everything that happened," which is less leading than providing specific and potentially leading reasons for disclosure (e.g., "It is really important that you tell me so I can put the suspect in jail"). Simply stating that "it is really important" is analogous to "placebic" requests that increase compliance without providing explicit justification (e.g., "May I use the Xerox machine because I have to make copies?" is more effective than "May I use the Xerox machine?"; Langer, Blank, & Chanowitz, 1978).

Interviewers should strive to ask children to describe individual abusive events (Lamb et al., 2008). When children narrate individual events, they are less likely to provide skeletal and generic reports and more likely to disclose idiosyncratic details, such as interruptions (e.g., the perpetrator stopped because a parent was heard coming home). Idiosyncratic details are harder to attribute to some sort of adult coaching. On the other hand, interviewers should avoid asking children to estimate the number of times abuse occurred or temporal information about the abuse, because this is likely to make true reports more difficult to distinguish from false reports. Children have difficulty providing numerical estimates in general. Children may also have particular difficulty with time and number if they are asked to recall incidents that occurred on multiple occasions over a long period of time (Lyon & Saywitz, 2006). Moreover, children's responses to direct questions about time and number are likely to be cursory whether their report is true or false.

It is also useful to ask children what occurred before and after the abusive contact. An adult who suggestively questions a child or who coaches the child to make a false report is likely to focus on eliciting the abusive act itself rather than the context in which the abuse occurred. Children who experienced sexual abuse are frequently able to provide information about the perpetrator's preparatory actions (e.g., closing the bedroom door), the immediate after-effects of the abuse (e.g., washing up, difficulty in falling asleep), and the perpetrator's efforts to conceal what occurred (e.g., telling the child not to tell). Interviewers can also ask more direct questions about what the child and the suspect did following the abuse (e.g., "What did he do after [the touching]?" "What did you do after he left?") and what children thought or felt about the incident (e.g., "How did you feel when he x?" "What did you think when he x?"). Children who report multiple episodes of abuse can be asked about their thoughts and feelings during early and later abuse incidents. This may elicit children's naïveté regarding the perpetrator's intentions initially and their fearful expectations on later occasions. Children are often remarkably articulate with respect to describing their emotional and physical reactions to abuse (Lyon, Scurich, Choi, Handmaker, & Blank, in press).

Children often report that genital touching occurred during caretaking, such as toileting or bathing, which may make it difficult to distinguish between abusive and innocuous touch. In addition to asking questions about what the suspect said about the touching, which might support sexual intent, the interviewer can ask the child about what occurs when others bathe or care for the child, which may enable the interviewer to determine if the suspect's actions were innocent or abusive.

Interviewers can better understand the social and emotional pressures on the child by inquiring into the child's prior disclosures and the child's reasons for disclosing (or for not disclosing sooner; Hershkowitz, Lanes, & Lamb, 2007). Information about the disclosure can be elicited by continuing to ask "what happened next" questions until children report telling another person (Hershkowitz et al., 2007), or the interviewer can ask the child in a more focused manner "Who did you tell?" and "What did you say to them?" The interviewer should also ask the child about the disclosure recipient's reactions ("What did she do/say when you told her?") and what the disclosure recipient has told the child about talking to the interviewer ("What did your mom tell you about talking to me?"). The interviewer should also ask the child what the parent and other interested adults have said about the alleged perpetrator ("What has x said about y?").

The responses of the people to whom the child disclosed are very important. Children, particularly young children, are likely to disclose abuse first to a parent (Kogan, 2004; Hershkowitz et al., 2007). Children are less likely to disclose and more likely to recant when nonoffending parents refuse to believe that abuse occurred or otherwise fail to support the allegation (Lawson & Chaffin, 1992; Malloy, Lyon, & Quas, 2007). On the other hand, children's reports are often doubted because of the assertion that a parent is influencing the child to make a false claim of abuse. Hence, the parent's reaction can play an important role in determining if the child's report is consistent over time. The interviewer can also ask the child what the perpetrator has said about others (including caregivers) and about the abuse, as this may reveal threats and other inducements to keep the abuse a secret and thus help to explain delays and inconsistencies in the child's report.

In order to distinguish between events the child reports because he or she has heard about events from others and events the child has actually experienced, the interviewer can ask the child "how do you know" questions. These are called "source monitoring" questions. Although these questions are very difficult for young preschoolers, who have limited abilities to identify the source of their beliefs (Gopnik & Graf, 1988), older children can report whether they actually saw or merely heard about events. Indeed, the Sam Stone study (Leichtman & Ceci, 1995), which documented high rates of false reports in preschoolers exposed to both repeated suggestive questioning about and negative stereotyping of a stranger who briefly visited the classroom, found that the rate of false reports decreased from 72% to 44% among three- to four- year olds and from approximately 30% to 10% among five- to six- year olds when children were asked "Did you *see* Sam Stone rip the book?" and "Did you *see* Sam Stone soil the teddy bear?" (see also Poole & Lindsay, 2001).

Some source monitoring questions may be less effective, such as questioning whether a recipient "told" the child what happened (Bruck, Melnyk, & Ceci, 2000). Young children often confuse "tell" and "ask" (Walker, 1999) and may not understand the implication of a question such as "Did your mother tell you what to say?" The question implies that the mother coached the child, but speaking literally, a mother who tells the child to "tell the truth" or "tell them what really happened" is telling the child "what to say." Moreover, "how do you know" questions are preferable to "did you see" questions insofar as the latter are yes–no questions and therefore less likely to elicit less accurate responses.

All of these inquiries enable the interviewer to test alternative hypotheses regarding the child's actual experiences. Asking about others' reactions, for example, helps the interviewer explore the possibility that the child is either alleging or denying abuse because of pressures from adults close to the child. Suggestibility researchers have argued that "[w]hen an interviewer avoids confirmatory biases by posing and testing alternative hypotheses, the suggestive techniques do not seem to result in as many serious problems" (Bruck, Ceci, & Melnyk, 1997, p. 304). We would caution, however, that the questions designed to test alternative hypotheses should themselves be worded in as open-ended a fashion as possible (e.g., "Tell me about a time your mom gave you a bath" and "What did your mom say about talking to the police?"). Questions that are sometimes recommended to test one's hypotheses about the child's abuse report (e.g., "Who else beside your teacher touched your private parts? Did your mommy touch them, too?"; Bruck, Ceci, & Hembrooke, 1998) risk eliciting inaccurate responses because of their directness.

The most widely researched guideline for conducting child interviews is the NICHD investigative interview protocol (Lamb et al., 2008). Under the NICHD protocol, child interviewers administer scripted interview instructions, rapport building questions, and nonleading allegation questions. International research testing the NICHD protocol demonstrates its superiority to nonprotocol interviews (Lamb et al., 2008). For example, interviewers using the NICHD protocol use at least three times more open-ended and approximately half as many option-posing and suggestive prompts as they do without the protocol, considering comparable incidents involving children of the same age (Lamb et al., 2008).

The Ten-Step interview (Lyon, 2005) is a modified and simplified version of the NICHD protocol. Because of research warning that children may overuse responses they are taught are acceptable (such as the "I don't know" response; Gee et al., 1999; Saywitz & Moan-Hardie, 1994), the Ten-Step includes a counterexample for each instruction. For example, the "I don't know" instruction reinforces both a "don't know" response (to "What is my dog's name?") and a responsive answer (to "Do you have a dog?"). Because of research demonstrating that eliciting a promise to tell the truth from children increases children's honesty (Evans & Lee, 2010; Lyon & Dorado, 2008; Lyon et al., 2008; Talwar et al., 2002, 2004), the Ten-Step includes the promise.

In sum, children's disclosures of sexual abuse can be highly probative evidence that abuse occurred. Laboratory research supports the conclusion that if a child discloses genital touching in response to free recall questions about interactions with an individual, this is strong evidence that such touching occurred. Even "yes" responses to recognition questions that would be considered inappropriately leading by many researchers (such as questioning with the assistance of an anatomically correct doll) are often strong evidence, but the strength of the evidence diminishes as the suggestiveness increases and the age of the child decreases. Laboratory research also supports the conclusion that interviewers can elicit more accurate reports from children with the use of open-ended questions, interview instructions (including a promise to tell the truth), and narrative practice rapport-building. Interview protocols that incorporate these elements are therefore likely to produce more accurate reports, in particular by reducing the likelihood that a false allegation will either be created or perpetuated by poor interviewing.

DIFFERENCES BETWEEN OUR ANALYSIS AND HERMAN (2009)

Our conclusions are quite different than one put forward by Herman (2009), who argues that "[f]alse positive error rates in forensic interviews are too high for these interviews to be used as the basis for making validity judgments about children's reports of CSA" (p. 261). Herman (2009) describes a study by Hershkowitz and colleagues (2007) that found that although trained evaluators exhibited "fairly high rates of overall accuracy compared with the accuracy of clinical judgements in other areas of psychology and medicine" when considering true and false reports elicited using the NICHD protocol, they were unable to discriminate between true and false reports elicited with nonprotocol interviews (p. 253). Moreover, for both the NICHD protocol and the nonprotocol interviews, evaluators judged a large percentage of the false disclosures as true.

The problem with Herman's analysis is that the study by Hershkowitz and colleagues (2007) did *not* assess the probative value of disclosures of sexual abuse. Rather, they looked at whether true disclosures could be distinguished from false disclosures. This is an important issue, but it begs the question of whether disclosures increase the likelihood that abuse occurred. The Hershkowitz and colleagues (2007) study *only* examined cases in which a child disclosed sexual abuse. It then selected equal numbers of true and false disclosures for both the NICHD protocol and nonprotocol interviews. In order to assess the probative value of a disclosure, however, it is important to recognize that a disclosure is itself highly probative of abuse and that good interviewing is less likely to elicit false disclosures than bad interviewing.

An analogy might help to make this point more clear. Imagine someone claimed that DNA tests are worthless because true matches look the same as false matches. In true matches, the perpetrator really did contribute the DNA sample found at the scene of the crime. In false matches, the perpetrator didn't contribute the DNA sample found at the scene of the crime, but the test result is positive; perhaps there was a lab error (for example, we don't have the perpetrator's actual DNA) or perhaps we have a random match (in which someone with DNA identical to the perpetrator actually contributed the DNA sample found at the scene of the crime). If the study compared true matches to false matches, they would be very difficult (perhaps impossible) to distinguish. Indeed, if they are both actual matches, they should look identical. It would be wrong, however, to conclude that a DNA match means nothing. Rather, one would ask what is the likelihood of a true match compared to a false match? As long as true matches are much more likely than false matches, then a match is highly probative evidence.

Imagine a second DNA study was conducted following the implementation of improved procedures that ensured that the only false matches are random matches. But again, if the study compared true matches to false matches, they would be difficult, if not impossible, to distinguish. It would be wrong, however, to conclude that improved procedures are ineffective. Rather, one would ask whether the number of true matches compared to the number of false matches increased, thus increasing the probative value of a match.

A disclosure of sexual abuse is analogous to a match. A true disclosure is like a true match. A false disclosure is like a false match. There is good evidence that disclosure of sexual abuse is much more likely to be true than false and that improving interviewing can reduce the likelihood of false disclosures. But these virtues are not detectable if one only compares true and false disclosures.

A second problem with using the Hershkowitz and colleagues (2007) study to argue that child interviews are not helpful is that the determination of whether sexual abuse occurred is not solely based on the word of the child. Herman (2009) is careful to make this point with respect to the existence of corroborative evidence, including perpetrator confessions, medical evidence, and eyewitness reports. However, he argues that unless this kind of corroborative evidence (which he calls "hard" evidence) is present, a child's disclosure (which he calls "soft" evidence) cannot suffice to substantiate an abuse report.

In a supplemental technical document (available on the Internet), Herman (2008) also acknowledges that evaluators

> might have interviews with the alleged perpetrator and other parties involved in the case, data about the context and manner in which the concern about possible sexual abuse first arose, data regarding the number of people who had talked with the child about suspected abuse before the recorded interviews occurred, as well as other case history information. It is possible that access to this additional information could improve decision accuracy across all cases...

Herman (2009) groups this type of information with the child's disclosure, thus categorizing it all as "soft" (p. 247). However, this is precisely the kind of information that can enable an interviewer to determine the risk that the child's prior and current disclosure are the product of suggestion, coercion, or insincerity. Moreover, as we have emphasized, the child interview itself should inquire into the child's initial disclosure and the pressures that have been placed on the child to disclose or not to disclose.

DISCUSSION

Bayesian approaches, if correctly understood, can help us understand the probative value of evidence. Children's disclosures of genital touch often constitute strong evidence that touching did in fact occur. If a grade-school child recalls genital touch in response to free recall questions, this is particularly strong evidence. More suggestive questions asked of younger children have less probative value.

Happily, researchers have moved beyond identifying methods that undermine children's accuracy and have developed positive prescriptions for effective interviewing. Interviews that utilize the tools incorporated into the NICHD structured interview protocol, including instructions, narrative practice rapport building, and open-ended questions regarding abuse, will lead to more accurate and complete reports. Furthermore, these methods can be further improved through the use of instructions with counterexamples and a promise to tell the truth (e.g., in the Ten-Step interview). Interviewers may elicit information from the child that helps the interviewer assess the likelihood that the child's report has been distorted by others, including the suspect and prior recipients of the child's disclosure.

NOTES

1. The reader might want to work through some more examples. Ten percent is equivalent to 10: (100–10), or 10:90, or 1:9. Twenty-fiver percent is equivalent to 25: (100–25) or 25:75 or 1:3. Seventy-five percent is equivalent to 75: (100–75) or 75:25, or 3:1.

2. To convert odds back to percentages we divide the first number in the odds ratio (20) by the sum of the first and the second numbers in the odds ratio (20 + 19). That is, we divide 20 by (20 + 19), which is 20/39, or 51%. Again, the reader will want to try some more examples. 1:1 converts to 50% because 1 divided by (1+1) is 1/2 or 50%. 2:1 converts to 67% because 2 divided by (2 + 1) is 2/3 or 67%. 100:1 converts to 99% because 100 divided by (100+1) is 99/100 or 99%.

3. The false positive rate is the inverse of the true negative rate; their sum equals 100%. If the child is not abused and the evidence is absent, this is a true negative. If the child is not abused and the evidence is present, this is a false positive. Hence, the likelihood that the evidence is present plus the likelihood that the evidence is absent will be 100%. If the true negative rate is 75%, the false positive rate is 25%.

REFERENCES

Bolstad, W. M. (2007). *Introduction to Bayesian statistics.* Hoboken, NJ: Wiley.

Bridges, A., Faust, D., & Ahern, D. (2009). Methods for the identification of sexually abused children. In K. Kuehnle & M. Connell (Eds.), *The evaluation of child sexual abuse allegations: A comprehensive guide to assessment and testimony* (pp. 21–47). Hoboken, NJ: John Wiley & Sons.

Brown, D., & Lamb, M. E. (2009). Forensic interviews with children: A two-way street: Supporting interviewers in adhering to best practice recommendations and enhancing children's capabilities in forensic interviews. In K. Kuehnle & M. Connell (Eds.), *The evaluation of child sexual abuse allegations: A comprehensive guide to assessment and testimony* (pp. 299–325). Hoboken, NJ: John Wiley & Sons.

Bruck, M., & Ceci, S. J. (1996). Issues in the scientific validation of interviews with young children. *Monographs of the Society for Research in Child Development, 61,* 204–214 (4–5, serial no. 248).

Bruck, M., & Ceci, S. J. (1999). The suggestibility of children's memory. *Annual Review of Psychology, 50,* 419–439.

Bruck, M., & Ceci, S. (2004). Forensic developmental psychology: Unveiling four common misconceptions. *Current Directions in Psychological Science, 13,* 229–232.

Bruck, M., Ceci, S. J., & Francouer, E. (2000). Children's use of anatomically detailed dolls to report genital touching in a medical examination: Developmental and gender comparisons. *Journal of Experimental Psychology: Applied, 6,* 74–83.

Bruck, M., Ceci, S. J., Francouer, E., & Renick, A. (1995). Anatomically detailed dolls do not facilitate preschoolers' reports of a pediatric examination involving genital touching. *Journal of Experimental Psychology: Applied, 1,* 95–109.

Bruck, M., Ceci, S. J., & Hembrooke, H. (1998). Reliability and credibility of young children's reports. *American Psychologist, 53*, 136–151.

Bruck, M., Ceci, S. J., & Melnyk, L. (1997). External and internal sources of variation in the creation of false reports in children. *Learning and Individual Differences, 9*, 289–316.

Carter, C., Bottoms, B. L., & Levine, M. (1996). Linguistic and socio-emotional influences on the accuracy of children's reports. *Law and Human Behavior, 20*, 335–358.

Cautilli, J. D., Riley-Tillman, T. C., Axelrod, S., & Hineline, P. (2005). The role of verbal conditioning in third generation behavior therapy. *The Behavior Analyst Today, 6*, 137–146.

Cordon, I. M., Saetermoe, C. L., & Goodman, G. S. (2005). Facilitating children's accurate responses: Conversational rules and interview style. *Applied Cognitive Psychology, 19*, 249–266.

Dale, P. S., Loftus, E. F., & Rathbun, L. (1978). The influence of the form of the question on the eyewitness testimony of preschool children. *Journal of Psycholinguistic Research, 74*, 269–277.

Davis, S. L., & Bottoms, B. L. (2002). Effects of social support on children's eyewitness reports: A test of the underlying mechanism. *Law and Human Behavior, 26*, 185–215.

Dent, H. R. (1982). The effects of interviewing strategies on the results of interviews with child witnesses. In A. Trankell (Ed.), *Reconstructing the past: The role of psychologists in criminal trials* (pp. 279–297). Stockholm, Sweden: Norstedt.

Dent, H. R. (1986). Experimental study of the effectiveness of different techniques of questioning child witnesses. *British Journal of Social and Clinical Psychology, 18*, 41–51.

Dent, H. R., & Stephenson, G. M. (1979). An experimental study of the effectiveness of different techniques of questioning child witnesses. *British Journal of Social and Clinical Psychology, 18*, 41–51.

Evans, A., & Lee, K. (2010). Promising to tell the truth makes 8- to 16-year-olds more honest. *Behavioral Sciences & the Law, 28*, 801–811.

Evett, I. W. (1995). Avoiding the transposed conditional. *Science & Justice, 35*, 127–131.

Faust, D., Bridges, A., & Ahern, D. (2009a). Methods for the identification of sexually abused children: Issues and needed features for abuse indicators. In K. Kuehnle & M. Connell (Eds.), *The evaluation of child sexual abuse allegations: A comprehensive guide to assessment and testimony* (pp. 3–19). Hoboken, NJ: John Wiley & Sons.

Faust, D., Bridges, A., & Ahern, D. (2009b). Methods for the identification of sexually abused children: Suggestions for clinical work and research. In K. Kuehnle & M. Connell (Eds.), *The evaluation of child sexual abuse allegations: A comprehensive guide to assessment and testimony* (pp. 49–66). Hoboken, NJ: John Wiley & Sons.

Finnila, K., Mahlberga, N., Santtilaa, P., & Niemib, P. (2003). Validity of a test of children's suggestibility for predicting responses to two interview situations differing in degree of suggestiveness. *Journal of Experimental Child Psychology, 85*, 32–49.

Garven, S., Wood, J. M., Malpass, R. S., & Shaw, J. S. (1998). More than suggestion: The effect of interviewing techniques from the McMartin preschool case. *Journal of Applied Psychology, 83,* 347–359.

Garven, S., Wood, J. M., Malpass, R. S., & Shaw, J. S. (2000). Allegations of wrongdoing: The effect of reinforcement on children's mundane and fantastic claims. *Journal of Applied Psychology, 85,* 38–49.

Geddie, L., Fradin, S., & Beer, J. (2000). Child characteristics which impact accuracy of recall and suggestibility in preschoolers: Is age the best predictor? *Child Abuse and Neglect, 24,* 223–235.

Gee, S., Gregory, M., & Pipe, M. E. (1999). "What colour is your pet dinosaur?" The impact of preinterview training and question type on children's answers. *Legal & Criminological Psychology, 4,* 111–128.

Goodman, G. S., & Aman, C. (1990). Children's use of anatomically detailed dolls to recount an event. *Child Development, 61,* 1859–1871.

Goodman, G. S., Bottoms, B. L., Schwartz-Kenney, B. M., & Rudy, L. (1991). Children's testimony about a stressful event: Improving children's reports. *Journal of Narrative and Life History, 1,* 69–99.

Goodman, G. S., & Quas, J. A. (2008). Repeated interviews and children's memory. It's more than just how many. *Current Directions in Psychological Science, 17,* 386–390.

Gopnik, A., & Graf, P. (1988). Knowing how you know: Young children's ability to identify and remember the sources of their beliefs. *Child Development, 59,* 1366–1371.

Heger, A., Ticson, L., Velasquez, O., & Bernier, R. (2002). Children referred for possible sexual abuse: Medical findings in 2384 children. *Child Abuse & Neglect, 26,* 645–659.

Herman, S. (2008). *Kuehnle/Connell book chapter supplement.* Retrieved from http://herman-research.blogspot.com/2008/03/next-two-subsections-roc-analysis-and_6775.html

Herman, S. (2009). Forensic child sexual abuse evaluations: Accuracy, ethics, and admissibility. In K. Kuehnle & M. Connell (Eds.), *The evaluation of child sexual abuse allegations: A comprehensive guide to assessment and testimony* (pp. 247–266). Hoboken, NJ: John Wiley & Sons.

Hershkowitz, I. (2009). Socioemotional factors in child sexual abuse investigations. *Child Maltreatment, 14,* 172–181.

Hershkowitz, I., Lanes, O., & Lamb, M. E. (2007). Exploring the disclosure of child sexual abuse with alleged victims and their parents. *Child Abuse & Neglect, 31,* 111–123.

Hutcheson, G. D., Baxter, J. S., Telfer, K., & Warden, D. (1995). Child witness statement quality: Question type and errors of omission. *Law and Human Behavior, 19,* 631–648.

Kaye, D. H., & Koehler, J. J. (1991). Can jurors understand probabilistic evidence? *Journal of the Royal Statistical Society A, 154,* 75–81.

Kogan, S. M. (2004). Disclosing unwanted sexual experiences: Results from a national sample of adolescent women. *Child Abuse & Neglect, 24,* 147–165.

Kuehnle, K., & Connell, M. (2009). *The evaluation of child sexual abuse allegations.* New York: Wiley.

Lamb, M. E., Hershkowitz, I., Orbach, Y., & Esplin, P. W. (2008). *Tell me what happened: Structured investigative interviews of child victims and witnesses*. West Sussex, England: Wiley.

Langer, E., Blank, A., & Chanowitz, B. (1978). The mindlessness of ostensibly thoughtful action: The role of placebic information in interpersonal interaction. *Journal of Personality and Social Psychology, 36*, 635–642.

LaRooy, D., Lamb, M. E., & Pipe, M. E. (2009). Repeated Interviewing: A critical evaluation of the risks and potential benefits. In K. Kuehnle & M. Connell (Eds.), *Critical issues in child sexual abuse assessment* (pp. 327–361). Hoboken, NJ: John Wiley & Sons.

Lawson, L., & Chaffin, M. (1992). False negatives in sexual abuse disclosure interviews: Incidence and influence of caretaker's belief in abuse in cases of accidental abuse discovery by diagnosis of STD. *Journal of Interpersonal Violence, 7*, 532–542.

Leichtman, M. D. & Ceci, S. J. (1995). The effects of stereotypes and suggestions on preschoolers' reports. *Developmental Psychology, 3*, 568–578.

Lyon, T. D. (1999). The new wave of suggestibility research: A critique. *Cornell Law Review, 84*, 1004–1087.

Lyon, T. D. (2005). *Ten step investigative interview*. Los Angeles: Author. Retrieved from http://works.bepress.com/thomaslyon/5/

Lyon, T. D., & Dorado, J. S. (2008). Truth induction in young maltreated children: The effects of oath-taking and reassurance on true and false disclosures. *Child Abuse & Neglect, 32*, 738–748.

Lyon, T. D., & Koehler, J. J. (1996). The relevance ratio: Evaluating the probative value of expert testimony in child sexual abuse cases. *Cornell Law Review, 82*, 43–78.

Lyon, T. D., Lamb, M. E., & Myers, J. (2009). Legal and psychological support for the NICHD interviewing protocol. *Child Abuse & Neglect, 33*, 71–74.

Lyon, T. D., Malloy, L. C., Quas, J. A., & Talwar, V. (2008). Coaching, truth induction, and young maltreated children's false allegations and false denials. *Child Development, 79*, 914–929.

Lyon, T. D., & Saywitz, K. J. (2006). From post-mortem to preventive medicine: Next steps for research on child witnesses. *Journal of Social Issues, 62*, 833–861.

Lyon, T. D., Scurich, N., Choi, K. Handmaker, S., & Blank, R. (in press). "How did you feel?" Increasing child sexual abuse witnesses' production of evaluative information. *Law & Human Behavior*.

Malloy, L. C., Lyon, T. D., & Quas, J. A. (2007). Filial dependency and recantation of child sexual abuse allegations. *Journal of the American Academy of Child and Adolescent Psychiatry, 46*, 162–170.

Memon, A. & Vartoukian, R. (1996). The effects of repeated questioning on young children's eyewitness testimony. *British Journal of Psychology, 87*, 403–415.

Moston, S. (1987). The suggestibility of children in interview studies. *First Language, 7*, 67–78.

Myers, J. E. B. (2005). *Myers on evidence in child, domestic, and elder abuse cases*. New York: Aspen Publishers.

Oates, K., & Shrimpton, S. (1991). Children's memories for stressful and non-stressful events. *Medical Science and Law, 31*, 4–10.

Ornstein, P. A., Gordon, B. N., & Larus, D. M., (1992). Children's memory for a personally experienced event: Implications for testimony. *Applied Cognitive Psychology, 6*, 49–60.

Perry, N., McAuliff, B., Tan, P., & Claycomb, C. (1995). When lawyers serve children: Is justice served? *Law and Human Behavior, 19*, 609–629.

Peters, W. W., & Nunez, N. (1999). Complex language and comprehension monitoring: Teaching child witnesses to recognize linguistic confusion. *Journal of Applied Psychology, 84*, 661–669.

Pipe, M. E., & Salmon, K. (2009). Dolls, drawing, body diagrams, and other props: Role of props in investigative interviews. In K. Kuehnle & M. Connell (Eds.), *The evaluation of child sexual abuse allegations: A comprehensive guide to assessment and testimony* (pp. 365–395). Hoboken, NJ: John Wiley & Sons.

Poole, D. A., & Lindsay, D. S. (2001). Children's eyewitness reports after exposure to misinformation from parents. *Journal of Experimental Psychology: Applied, 7*, 27–50.

Poole, D. A. & Wolfe, M. A. (2009). Child development: Normative sexual and nonsexual behaviors that may be confused with symptoms of sexual abuse. In K. Kuehnle & M. Connell (Eds.), *The evaluation of child sexual abuse allegations: A comprehensive guide to assessment and testimony* (pp. 101–128). Hoboken, NJ: John Wiley & Sons.

Roberts, K. P., Lamb, M. E., & Sternberg, K. J. (2004). The effects of rapport-building style on children's reports of a staged event. *Applied Cognitive Psychology, 18*, 189–202.

Saywitz, K. J., Goodman, G. S., Nicholas, G., & Moan, S. (1991). Children's memory of a physical examination involving genital touch: Implications for reports of child sexual abuse. *Journal of Consulting and Clinical Psychology, 5*, 682–691.

Saywitz, K. J., & Moan-Hardie, S. (1994). Reducing the potential for distortion of childhood memories. *Consciousness and Cognition, 3*, 257–293.

Saywitz, K. J., Snyder, L., & Nathanson, R. (1999). Facilitating the communicative competence of the child witness. *Applied Developmental Science, 3*, 58–68.

Schum, D. A., & Martin, A. W. (1982). Formal and empirical research on cascaded inference in jurisprudence. *Law & Society Review, 17*, 105–152.

Sternberg, K. J., Lamb, M. E., Hershkowitz, I., Yudilevitch, L., Orbach, Y., Esplin, P. W., et al. (1997). Effects of introductory style on children's abilities to describe experiences of sexual abuse. *Child Abuse and Neglect, 21*, 1133–1146.

Steward, M. S., Steward, D. S., Farquhar, L., Myers, J. E. B., Reinhart, M.,Welker, J., et al. (1996). Interviewing young children about body touch and handling. *Monographs of the Society for Research in Child Development, 61* (4–5, Serial No. 248).

Talwar, V., Lee, K., Bala, N., & Lindsay, R. C. L. (2002). Children's conceptual knowledge of lying and its relation to their actual behaviors: Implications for court competence examinations. *Law & Human Behavior, 26*, 395–415.

Talwar, V., Lee, K., Bala, N., & Lindsay, R. C. L. (2004). Children's lie-telling to conceal a parent's transgression: Legal implications. *Law & Human Behavior, 28*, 411–435.

Thompson, W. C., & Schumann, E. L. (1987). Interpretation of statistical evidence in criminaltrials: The prosecutors' fallacy and the defense attorney's fallacy. *Law and Human Behavior, 1*, 167–187.

Walker, A. G. (1999). *Handbook on questioning children: A linguistic perspective* (2nd ed.). Washington, DC: American Bar Association.

Warren, A, Hulse-Trotter, K., & Tubbs, E. (1991). Inducing resistance to suggestibility in children. *Law & Human Behavior, 15,* 273–285.

Wood, J. M. (1996). Weighing evidence in sexual abuse evaluations: An introduction to Bayes's Theorem. *Child Maltreatment, 1,* 25–36

AUTHOR NOTES

Thomas D. Lyon, PhD, JD, is the Judge Edward J. and Ruey L. Guirado Chair in Law and Psychology at the University of Southern California and researches child abuse and neglect, child witnesses, and domestic violence. He is the past-president of the American Psychological Association's Section on Child Maltreatment (Division 37) and a former member of the board of directors of the American Professional Society on the Abuse of Children.

Elizabeth C. Ahern, MA, is a PhD candidate in developmental psychology at the University of Southern California. She researches children's disclosure of maltreatment, truth induction methods, and emergent lie-telling ability. She is also a child interviewing specialist and conducts trainings on child interviewing.

Nicholas Scurich, MA, is a PhD candidate in quantitative psychology at the University of Southern California. He studies normative and descriptive models of juridical decision making.

CHALLENGES TO THE ACCURACY AND OBJECTIVITY OF CASE DECISION MAKING

Reliability of Professional Judgments in Forensic Child Sexual Abuse Evaluations: Unsettled or Unsettling Science?

MARK D. EVERSON
University of North Carolina at Chapel Hill, Chapel Hill, North Carolina, USA

JOSÉ MIGUEL SANDOVAL
Duke University, Durham, North Carolina, USA

NANCY BERSON, MARY CROWSON, and HARRIET ROBINSON
University of North Carolina at Chapel Hill, Chapel Hill, North Carolina, USA

In the absence of photographic or DNA evidence, a credible eyewitness, or perpetrator confession, forensic evaluators in cases of alleged child sexual abuse must rely on psychosocial or "soft" evidence, often requiring substantial professional judgment for case determination. This article offers a three-part rebuttal to Herman's (2009) argument that forensic decisions based on psychosocial evidence are fundamentally unreliable and that this conclusion represents settled science. The article also discusses the potentially adverse consequences of Herman's proposed reforms to forensic practice on child protection and prosecution efforts.

THE CASE AGAINST ESTABLISHED PRACTICE

"Hard" evidence that definitively proves or disproves the occurrence of abuse is uncommon in forensic assessments of child sexual abuse (CSA). In the absence of photographic or DNA evidence, a credible eyewitness, or a perpetrator confession, forensic evaluators typically must rely on an analysis of psychosocial or "soft" evidence, often requiring substantial professional judgment, for case determination. For example, such "soft" evidence might include the child's detailed, idiosyncratic descriptions of vaginal and anal penetration, school reports of behavior changes and sexual acting out, or prior, unsubstantiated claims of CSA by a second child against the alleged perpetrator. The use of psychosocial evidence in forensic CSA evaluations and investigations has long been viewed as essential practice (Faller, 2007). Recently, however, Herman (2009) has condemned the use of "soft" evidence in case decisions about sexual abuse, arguing that professional judgments derived from such evidence have been shown empirically to be unreliable. This article takes issue with the conclusions Herman draws from existing research as well as his call for "drastic reforms" of current forensic practice.

Several studies have examined the psychometric properties of professional judgments in forensic assessments of CSA (e.g., Horner, Guyer, & Kalter, 1992; Jackson & Nuttall, 1993). According to Herman (2005, 2009), such research consistently indicates that substantiation decisions that rely on clinical or professional judgment rather than "hard" evidence lack adequate reliability, validity, and accuracy. It is essential to note that much of the research Herman relied on for this conclusion about reliability, validity, and accuracy actually focused only on reliability, defined as the degree of agreement between evaluators examining the same evidence.

Assessment of the validity and accuracy of substantiation decisions requires knowledge of the truth of a maltreatment report. Several of the studies Herman cited used fictional case vignettes without a "true" abuse event, and the few studies using actual cases lacked a "gold standard" for knowing what really happened in a case. Reliability, however, does not require a "gold standard" classification of the case. One can observe that two evaluators disagree without knowing which one is correct. Since reliability is a minimal requirement for validity and accuracy, Herman was able to logically deduce that validity and accuracy in the studies was poor on the basis of their poor reliability. Furthermore, based on additional extrapolations from the reliability coefficients from these studies, Herman estimated the accuracy rates of evaluators correctly identifying valid versus false cases of CSA to be at most 76% across studies. Generalizing from these extrapolations to real forensic practice, Herman concluded that forensic evaluators are likely to be wrong in their substantiation decisions in at least 24% of cases—a rate appropriately described as unacceptably high.

In a chapter in Kuehnle and Connell's (2009) book, Herman (2009) highlighted the results of a decision making study among child abuse investigators in Israel (Hershkowitz, Fisher, Lamb, & Horowitz, 2007) as further evidence of the psychometric limitations of professional judgments about CSA. Forty-two experienced abuse investigators were asked to evaluate transcripts of actual investigative interviews with alleged child victims of sexual abuse and to make judgments about whether the allegations in each case were valid. Unlike prior studies of substantiation decisions, there was strong independent evidence that one-half of the cases were valid and one-half were false. Thus, Herman reasoned, the accuracy of the Israeli investigators in correctly categorizing the transcripts could be used to estimate the actual validity of professional decision making in CSA cases. Herman calculated the overall "hit rate" (the total percentage correct) to be 61%, only marginally better than the 50% rate expected by chance. Compared to the official categorization of cases as valid or false, these experienced investigators were wrong in the "substantiation" decisions in 39% of the cases—somewhat higher than Herman's (2005) minimal estimate of 24% of cases.

Citing the consistency of findings across empirical studies that "clinical judgments" in forensic evaluations lack reliability, accuracy, and validity, Herman (2009) has challenged the legitimacy and ethics of making decisions to substantiate CSA allegations without definitive "corroborating" evidence. Herman defines "corroborating evidence" narrowly, consistent with law enforcement usage to include only "hard evidence," with examples such as perpetrator confessions, significant medical findings, and photographs or videos of the abuse. He estimates that such evidence is available in approximately one-third of all forensic CSA evaluations and in half of all cases judged likely to be true by evaluators (see Olafson in this issue for a critique of these estimates). Herman is dismissive of attempts to make inferences about the validity of abuse allegations on the basis of soft or psychosocial evidence, including an analysis of the child's disclosure statement. He calls for "drastic reforms of current practice" (Herman, 2009, p. 259), including severe restrictions on the type of evidence considered in child protective services (CPS) and legal settings.

A THREE-PART REBUTTAL

This article refutes the central premise of Herman's argument that forensic CSA decisions made in the absence of definitive, corroborative evidence such as a confession, an eyewitness or videotapes of the abuse are fundamentally unreliable and that this conclusion represents settled science. Our response includes three parts. We begin by examining the research cited as evidence of the limited reliability and accuracy of substantiation decisions about CSA. We argue that these studies are unrepresentative of actual forensic practice, and that the study results cannot be generalized to the real world. Second, we offer a discussion of six design and analysis features that can be manipulated in decision-making studies to produce substantially different reliability estimates, depending on arbitrary decisions by the researcher. We offer this discussion as evidence that reliability estimates of professional judgment are in part an artifact of the research design and analysis. Third, we present the findings from a study of the reliability of professional judgments in CSA cases that demonstrates the impact of three of these factors on reliability estimates. Thus, we argue that (a) existing research is limited in its usefulness for assessing the reliability and validity of professional decision making in CSA assessments, and (b) the magnitude of reliability coefficients is dependent on arbitrary variations of study design, which limits the confidence we can place in their applicability to actual practice.

I. Examination Of Prior Research On Reliability

Herman's (2009) argument centers on seven published studies on the reliability (agreement between professionals examining the same evidence) and accuracy (the correct classification of cases as valid or invalid) of professional decisions in cases of alleged CSA. The seven studies are Finlayson and Koocher (1991); Hershkowitz and colleagues (2007); Horner and colleagues (1992); Horner, Guyer, and Kalter (1993); Jackson and Nuttall (1993); McGraw and Smith (1992); Realmuto, Jensen, and Wescoe (1990); and Realmuto and Wescoe (1992). Herman (2005) counts the Horner and colleagues' articles as a single study. An eighth study cited by Herman, an unpublished dissertation by Shumaker (2000), is omitted from this discussion due to its limited availability. The common methodology across studies involves asking professionals to rate the validity of a CSA allegation based on a review of a shared set of case facts. Professional judgments are reliable to the degree that professionals examining the same evidence arrive at similar conclusions about the validity of the allegation. Professional judgments are accurate to the degree that they agree with the "official" categorization of the case as true or untrue.

Herman (2005) was able to derive Cohen's kappa coefficients from data provided in five of these studies as estimates of the reliability of professional judgments. The kappas ranged from .08 to .42 with a mean of only .25. These kappas are generally considered to fall below acceptable levels for reliability (see, e.g., Fleiss, 1981; Landis & Koch, 1977). Herman (2009) described the Hershkowitz and colleagues (2007) study as the only study to date to directly assess the accuracy of professional judgments about the validity of CSA allegations. According to Herman, the reported hit rate of only 61% in correctly classifying cases as true or as false and the overall false positive rate of 44% serve as a serious indictment of the accuracy of current forensic practice. Taken together, these studies initially present a very unsettling picture of the reliability and accuracy of decisions in forensic child sexual abuse evaluations. However, on closer examination, it is clear that each study is limited in its generalizability to current forensic practice and therefore cannot be relied on to yield a meaningful estimate of the reliability of decision-making in the real world. Table 1 provides a description of the sample of professionals who served as research participants in each study. Only three of the studies examined judgments among professionals with specific training and experience in forensic assessments of child sexual abuse (Hershkowitz et al., 2007; McGraw & Smith, 1992; Realmuto & Wescoe, 1992). The research samples in the four remaining studies included psychologists "who worked with children" (Finlayson & Koocher 1991); professionals "with varying degrees of experience in child sexual abuse" (Jackson & Nuttall, 1993); a broad mix of mental health clinicians, trainees, and allied professionals (e.g., elementary school teachers and day care workers; Horner et al., 1992, 1993); and one "senior female child psychiatric resident" (Realmuto et al., 1990).

An even more critical factor limiting the generalizability of the cited research to actual forensic practice is the lack of ecological validity in all seven studies. Ecological validity refers to how closely the main methods and conditions of the study are realistic in approximating the real-life situation being investigated. In other words, the studies cited by Herman are ecologically valid and their results generalizable to current forensic practice *only* to the degree that the studies approximate current forensic practice. Although forensic practice varies somewhat by discipline, the most commonly endorsed and perhaps most widely used approach for assessing CSA allegations is the comprehensive forensic evaluation (CFE) model (American Professional Society on the Abuse of Children, 1997; Everson & Faller, this issue; Faller, 2007; Kuehnle, 1996, 1998). The CFE model therefore serves as an appropriate standard for assessments of the ecological validity of Herman's seven studies. Best practice methodology for the CFE model typically includes: the use of a broad range of information sources for a comprehensive search for evidence supporting or refuting the allegations, weighing substantive evidence based on the degree of independent corroboration, the testing of alternative hypotheses, and the construction of a case-specific narrative to account for the available evidence (Everson & Faller, this issue).

Table 1 describes the case information provided to research participants in each of the seven studies. Note that case material for five of the studies was unrealistically limited to a one- to two-page case summary, a written interview transcript, or a 20-minute video segment of an anatomical doll interview (Finlayson & Koocher, 1991; Hershkowitz et al., 2007; Jackson & Nuttall, 1993; Realmuto et al., 1990; Realmuto & Wescoe, 1992). For example, forensic evaluators in the Hershkowitz et al. (2007) study were asked to discriminate between true and false reports of CSA *solely* on the basis of a written transcript from a *single* child interview. Other case materials, including background and case history, prior statements by the child, history of behavior symptoms, medical records, and interviews with the alleged

TABLE 1 Summary of Published Studies on Reliability of Decision Making in CSA Cases

Study	Sample	Case material presented
Finlayson and Koocher (1991)	269 pediatric psychologists "who worked with children"	4 1/2 page case vignettes
Hershkowitz, Fisher, Lamb, and Horowitz (2007)	42 Israeli child forensic evaluators	Written transcripts from 24 child interviews
Horner, Guyer, and Kalter (1992, 1993)	129 mental health clinicians, trainees, and allied professionals (e.g., teachers, child care providers)	Comprehensive oral summary of 1 case involving a 3-year-old girl in contested custody proceedings
Jackson and Nuttall (1993)	656 professionals "with varying degrees of experience in CSA," recruited from national directories of clinical social workers, pediatricians, psychiatrists, and psychologists	16 one-page case vignettes
McGraw and Smith (1992)	Undisclosed number of CPS workers from the Boulder County, Colorado, DSS who investigated 18 cases of alleged sexual abuse in 1986 and 1987	Case files for 18 children involved in contested divorce or custody proceedings
Realmuto, Jensen, and Wescoe (1990)	1 "senior female child psychiatric resident"	20 minute anatomical doll interview of 15 children, ages 4–8, conducted by the psychiatric resident
Realmuto and Wescoe (1992)	14 professionals with at least 10 years of experience with CSA cases (3 pediatricians, 3 child psychologists, 3 social workers, 3 attorneys, and 2 psychologists)	20 minute anatomical doll interview of 13 children, ages 3 1/2–7

offender and various collaterals that are typically available in comprehensive forensic evaluations, were deliberately withheld. There was also no video recording to allow direct observation of body language, demeanor, or a host of other verbal and nonverbal cues that might aid their assessment. There was no opportunity for follow-up questions by the forensic evaluators or a follow-up interview if the child's statement was unclear or inconsistent.

As other examples of research with limited ecological validity, professionals participating in the two Realmuto studies (Realmuto et al., 1990; Realmuto & Wescoe, 1992) were required to judge the validity of abuse allegations exclusively on the statements and behavior of children in 20 minute anatomical doll interviews. Increasing the impossibility of this exercise, the university institutional review board (IRB) overseeing the research had imposed significant restrictions on the types of questions interviewers in the 20 minute doll interviews were permitted to ask. Needless to say, the methodology employed in the Realmuto studies bears little resemblance to any recognizable form of current forensic assessment.

In contrast, the range of information available to participants in the McGraw and Smith (1992) and Horner et al. (1992, 1993) studies was comprehensive in nature and included case information collected in actual CPS investigations (McGraw & Smith, 1992) or in a formal forensic evaluation (Horner et al., 1992, 1993). However, given the substantial evolution of forensic practice since the mid-1990s, especially in approaches to child forensic interviewing, it is questionable whether CPS investigations conducted in 1986–1987 and a forensic evaluation conducted in the early 1990s are representative of current practice in comprehensive forensic investigations or evaluations.

Finally, the Horner and colleagues (1992, 1993) research faces another ecological validity challenge, one that is shared by the rest of Herman's seven studies, except for McGraw and Smith (1992). In Horner and colleagues (1992, 1993) and the other studies, the research participants were asked to rate the credibility or validity of an abuse allegation as part of a research exercise. It is important to recognize that the professional judgments that such ratings reflect are not equivalent to case decisions in actual forensic evaluations. Unlike the anonymous, comparatively frivolous ratings in research exercises, case decisions are public, have potentially life-changing implications for many of the parties involved, and may require defense in legal proceedings. As a result, actual case decisions are likely to be more deliberative, cautious, and constrained by the strength of legally defensible evidence than are professional judgments in research exercises. Professional judgments assessed in such exercises may provide insights into predispositions and biases and thus have utility, but their direct generalizability to actual public case decisions may be limited.

In conclusion, the seven studies Herman (2005, 2009) relies on to justify his condemnation of forensic assessment are severely limited individually and as a group in their generalizability to current accepted practice and in particular to evaluations employing best practice standards of the comprehensive forensic evaluation model (Everson & Faller, this issue). Simply put, Herman's (2005, 2009) conclusions about the reliability, validity, and accuracy of forensic CSA evaluations, including his estimate of a 24% error rate in substantiation decisions, are empirically unfounded.

II. Design Features that Affect Assessments of Reliability

Definitive reliability estimates for professional judgments in CSA evaluations are illusive. Reliability estimates may vary widely across studies, depending on several design features. In fact, reliability estimates can be significantly manipulated by implementation of any of the following design options:

Provision of a Comprehensive Versus Narrow Range of Case Information

Whether case decisions are based on a comprehensive or narrow range of case information is a paramount issue in substantiation research. As discussed, making a substantiation decision solely on the basis of psychosocial evidence of limited source and scope (e.g., a 20-minute doll interview) is unrealistic and would likely be considered a breach of accepted practice. Case evidence of such limited scope precludes evaluators from using their full complement of decision-making criteria, likely resulting in more frequent inconclusive decisions. Forcing judgments on the basis of inadequate information encourages the use of subjective factors as a substitute for case facts, likely increasing the frequency of case disagreements.

Degree of Case Ambiguity

Perhaps the single most effective way of manipulating the level of agreement in reliability studies is to manipulate the case evidence. Agreement will be high to the degree that there is compelling evidence supporting a single hypothesis in the case. As evidence is added that supports alternative hypotheses, case ambiguity and professional disagreements may increase. Researchers can therefore manipulate the strength of reliability coefficients in decision-making studies by selecting actual cases or writing case scenarios that support multiple, plausible hypotheses to explain the allegations.

The Finlayson and Koocher (1991) findings provide an example of this point. They asked pediatric psychologists to rate the likelihood of CSA having occurred in four clinical vignettes that involved identical child and family variables but varying symptom patterns. As more compelling evidence in support of an abuse hypothesis was added to the case scenarios, agreement among the participating psychologists as to whether sexual abuse had occurred increased from 70% that it had not to 98% that it had. The Finlayson and Koocher findings suggest that, with a little pilot testing, one can develop scenarios to produce virtually any level of agreement desired.

Varying the Definition of "Substantiated"

The definition of the term "substantiated," as it applies to CPS investigations of abuse, varies across states (U.S. Department of Health and Human Services, 2003). Part of the variation involves the level of evidence or certainty required to substantiate an allegation. In 19 states, CPS agencies use a "some credible evidence" or "probable cause" standard of certainty in dispositional decisions, while 23 states require a higher "preponderance of evidence" standard of certainty. Although it is unclear whether differing standards of proof affect CPS practice (Levine, 1998), similar differentiation is possible in research, with likely implications for both the proportion of cases that are rated as substantiated and the level of agreement between study participants. The broader definition, depending on how it is operationalized, will be associated with a greater proportion of cases categorized as "substantiated" and therefore increased agreement in valid CSA cases.

Varying the Definition of "Unsubstantiated"

In 23 states, CPS defines "unsubstantiated" broadly in terms of "insufficient evidence to substantiate" (U.S. Department of Human Services, 2003). By this definition, unsubstantiated is a catch-all category that includes all cases that fail to meet the substantiation threshold. Twenty-six states, however, define unsubstantiated more narrowly as cases in which abuse has been ruled out. This stricter definition limits the number of cases classified as unsubstantiated and often includes the creation of at least one additional category (sometimes labeled as "indicated") for cases that are neither substantiated nor unsubstantiated. In reliability research, the choice of which definition of unsubstantiated is used can affect outcomes. The broader catch-all definition will likely result in a higher proportion of cases rated as unsubstantiated, with a subsequent decrease in agreement in valid CSA cases.

Provision of Decision Making Criteria

The accuracy of decision making in CSA cases involves at least two components: (a) the validity of the substantiation criteria used to categorize allegations as true or not true, and (b) the accuracy of the evaluator in applying the substantiation criteria. An evaluator can reach an erroneous decision in a CSA assessment through the use of invalid criteria for judging the trueness of the allegation or by misapplying valid criteria. An example of the use of an invalid substantiation criterion is the evaluator who concludes a seven-year-old is fabricating her report of fondling because she does not exhibit visible signs of distress during disclosure. An example of the second type of error is the evaluator who correctly believes that substantial consistency across descriptions of the same abusive event is a characteristic of most true cases but who concludes a case is false because a five-year-old child is "inconsistent" in answering the question "How many times did it happen?" In one interview the child answers "50 times" and in another, "100 times."

Most reliability studies fail to distinguish between the two components. One way to more accurately assess the professional judgment component is to provide the substantiation criteria to be used by all evaluators and to assess variation among evaluators using the same criteria. In other words, the criteria are held constant. This was done as part of an evaluation of an in-service training course on CSA investigations for California CPS workers (Parry, 2009). As a final assessment, course participants were asked to make judgments about whether abuse had occurred in four written scenarios involving CSA allegations based on the decision-making criteria they were taught in the course. The percent of participants agreeing with the official case designation as abuse or no abuse was 90% or higher for each scenario. Kappa statistics of .64 and above also indicated excellent agreement. These findings suggest that substantial agreement in professional judgments about the validity of CSA allegations can be achieved if the same criteria for decision making are used across professionals rather than being allowed to vary idiosyncratically by professional.

Exclusion of Undecided or "No Judgment Possible" Cases

In the real world of CPS investigations and forensic assessments, many cases end with an inconclusive finding. There is insufficient evidence for the evaluator to make a judgment that abuse likely occurred or did not occur (or, more precisely, the evaluator's substantiation criteria are inadequate, given the available evidence, for categorizing the case). CPS agencies in 14 states recognize these cases as a separate formal category, usually termed "unable to determine or complete" (U.S. Department of Human Services, 2003). Such cases are sometimes referred for additional assessment or flagged for future monitoring. Oates and colleagues (1999) reported a 21% rate of "inconclusive" cases in a 551 case sample of Denver CPS investigations of CSA. Similarly, 21 out of 104 comprehensive forensic CSA evaluations conducted in a specialized assessment program over a 10-year period by the current authors were classified as no judgment possible (NJP).

Research participants who are asked to rate the credibility of a case on a Likert scale and are not given an explicit NJP category to choose typically rate NJP/indeterminate cases in the midrange of scores. In research on the reliability of professional judgments, NJP/indeterminate case decisions are usually interpreted as a decision against substantiation and are therefore included in the unsubstantiation count (e.g., Hershkowitz et al., 2007). Alternatively, an NJP decision can be viewed as an abstention or nonvote and excluded from both substantiation and nonsubstantiation tallies. Omitting NJP/indeterminate case decisions from agreement/disagreement calculations and limiting assessments of the reliability of professional judgments to cases in which professional judgments are actually made will likely improve both the strength and accuracy of reliability estimates.

III. Impact of Variations in Design Features

Next, we will describe the results of a study that manipulated three of these design features to assess their impact on reliability estimates. A fourth

TABLE 2 Demographic Characteristics of Overall Sample and Three Decision Exercise Subsamples

	Overall sample		Decision Exercise Subsamples					
			Case summaries		Mock evaluation		Record review	
Demographic	n	%	n	%	n	%	n	%
Sample Source								
State Conference/Workshops	315	56.1	124	100	124	100	67	21.4
National Conference	246	43.9	0	0	0	0	246	78.6
Professional Position								
CPS	194	34.6	61	49.2	13	10.5	120	38.3
MH	137	24.4	8	6.4	92	74.2	37	11.8
LE	84	14.9	18	14.5	0	0	66	21.1
ATT	44	7.8	17	12.7	0	0	27	8.6
CFE	23	4.1	4	3.2	7	5.6	12	3.8
CFI	79	14.1	16	12.9	12	9.7	51	16.3
Experience								
0–2 yrs	267	24.5	98	42.0	15	13.4	46	18.5
3–10 yrs	531	48.8	113	48.0	52	46.4	130	52.4
>10 yrs	290	26.7	24	10.2	45	40.2	72	29.0
Gender								
Male	120	21.5	20	16.1	25	20.5	75	23.9
Female	459	78.5	104	83.9	97	79.5	238	76.0

Note: CPS = child protective services, MH = mental health, LE = law enforcement, ATT = attorney, CFE = child forensic evaluator, CFI = child forensic interviewer. The case summary, mock evaluation, and record review subsamples shared little to no overlap in participants.

feature, provision of a broad range of case information for decision making, was held constant to approximate actual forensic practice. Study participants included 561 professionals active in the field of child maltreatment. As shown in Table 2, they included CPS workers (CPS); child therapists and other mental health professionals (MH); law enforcement officers (LE); attorneys, most of whom were prosecutors (ATT); child forensic evaluators (CFE); and child forensic interviewers (CFI). In order to broaden sample representativeness, study participants were recruited from three sources: a plenary session of a national child abuse conference, a state child abuse conference, and 12 continuing education workshops throughout the state of North Carolina. Estimated participation rates included 70% of those attending the national conference plenary session, 48% of professionals receiving a copy of research materials at the state conference, and 95–100% of professionals attending in-state trainings.

Each study participant completed one of three forensic decision-making exercises that involved rating the likely validity of one or two cases of alleged child sexual abuse after reviewing a set of case materials. Four "fictional" cases were used. They were developed to reflect varying levels of case ambiguity and, in order to increase realism, were based loosely on actual cases or were derived from the authors' extensive assessment experience. (See Everson & Sandoval, 2011, for a more complete description of sample recruitment and study methodology.) Descriptions of the decision exercises follow.

DECISION EXERCISES

Record Review Exercise (n = 313). This exercise was designed as a mock case record review based in part on an actual case of a 4-year-old who made allegations that she had been fondled by her 13-year-old cousin. The "record" provided to participants was a detailed, eight-page, single-spaced summary of the initial allegation report, case background, medical examination, collateral interviews, and interviews with the alleged perpetrator. It also included a partial transcript of a forensic interview with the alleged victim. Participants were asked to rate the likely validity of the allegation on a 10-point rating scale.

Mock Evaluation (n = 124). As part of a two-day workshop on forensic evaluations in cases of alleged abuse, participants spent three hours working in multidisciplinary groups of four on a mock evaluation based loosely on a real case of alleged abuse. The case involved allegations of sexual abuse of a four-year-old by her biological father, resulting in a divorce and legal battles over visitation. The small groups were given the task of designing and conducting a forensic evaluation in the allotted time with the goal of producing a set of written conclusions and recommendations. The evaluation was an iterative process in which groups requested and reviewed specific data packets (e.g., CPS records, medical files, interviews with child) before asking for additional data packets as the case unfolded. Up to 30 different data packets were available for review. After the groups had completed the exercise, and prior to a plenary group discussion of the case, participants were asked to set aside their group's conclusions about the validity of the case and to complete ratings of what they believed "in their heart of hearts." Specifically, participants were asked to rate the likely validity of the allegation on a scale of one to seven.

Case Summaries (n = 124). Study participants in this exercise reviewed two different case summaries. Both involved preschool-age girls as alleged victims of fondling, one by her babysitter's 14-year-old son, the other by the girl's maternal grandfather. A two to three page summary was provided for each case that included a partial transcript of the child's statement, interviews with the child's mother and with the alleged abuser, and a summary of the medical findings. Participants were asked to rate the likely validity of the allegation in each case on a 10-point scale.

Operationalization of Design Features

From the six design features described earlier, three were chosen for study based on feasibility and ease of implementation. The three features and their method of operationalization are described next.

Degree of Case Ambiguity. Case ambiguity was varied across the four cases by manipulating the consistency of the psychosocial evidence supporting one, or more than one, possible explanation for the abuse allegations. Three levels of case ambiguity were included: *minimal ambiguity*—clear evidence abuse likely occurred (case summary 1) and clear evidence abuse likely did not occur (case summary 2), *moderate ambiguity*—some contradictory evidence, and *substantial ambiguity*—significant contradictory evidence regarding whether abuse occurred.

Varying the Definition of "Substantiation." Two definitions of "substantiation" were compared: a credible evidence standard of certainty and a preponderance of evidence standard of certainty. Operationalization involved the use of differing scoring protocols for categorizing cases as substantiated or not substantiated on the basis of the validity rating assigned by study participants. As shown in Table 3, the scoring protocols used differing cut-points for dichotomizing the 7-point or 10-point scale into "substantiated" and "unsubstantiated" categories. Specifically, a rating of 5, 6, or 7 on the 7-point mock evaluation rating was defined as "substantiated" using the credible evidence standard, while a rating of 1, 2, 3, or 4 was defined as "unsubstantiated." In contrast, substantiation was defined more narrowly for

TABLE 3 Scoring Protocols for Operationalizing "Varying Definition of Substantiated" and "NJP Excluded" Design Features

	7 Point Validity Rating Scale						
	Very likely untrue 1	2	3	4	5	6	Very likely true 7
Preponderance Standard	U	U	U	U	U	S	S
Credible Standard	U	U	U	U	S	S	S
NJP Excluded	U	U	U	—	S	S	S

	10 Point Validity Rating Scale									
	Very likely untrue 1	2	3	4	5	6	7	8	9	Very likely true 10
Preponderance Standard	U	U	U	U	U	U	U	S	S	S
Credible Standard	U	U	U	U	U	U	S	S	S	S
NJP Excluded	U	U	U	U	—	—	S	S	S	S

Note: NJP = no judgment possible, S = scored as substantiated, U = scored as unsubstantiated, — = Omitted from analysis.

the preponderance of evidence standard, with a cut-point between 5 and 6 so that ratings of 6 or greater were categorized as substantiated while 1 to 5 were labeled unsubstantiated. Table 3 provides a similar comparison of the cut-points for the credible and preponderance standards scenarios for the 10-point record review and case summary ratings.

Exclusion of Undecided or NJP Cases. The scoring protocol for this design feature designated the midpoint of each validity rating scale as the NJP/indeterminate category. As a result, ratings of 4 on the 7-point validity scale and 5 or 6 on the 10-point scale were excluded from reliability calculations, effectively treating midpoint ratings as missing data.

Reliability findings

Table 4 provides a summary of the kappa and percentage agreement reliability coefficients for the four cases. These coefficients reflect the number of study participants in agreement on case validity ratings for each scoring protocol. There are several findings of note:

1. As expected, reliability coefficients varied widely across cases and scoring protocols, with kappas ranging from .00 to .97 and percentage agreements ranging from 49% to 99% (Randolph, 2008). For comparison purposes, adequate reliability was defined as a percentage of agreement of 86% or higher and a kappa of .50 or higher (the mid-moderate range of agreement using the Landis and Koch [1977] guidelines for kappa interpretation). Adequate to excellent reliability was therefore obtained for 6 of the 12 scoring protocol-by-case combinations, while

TABLE 4 Impact of Design Features on Kappa and Percentage Agreement Reliability Coefficients

Decision exercise	Degree of case ambiguity	Preponderance of evidence %	k	Credible evidence %	k	NJP cases excluded %	k	Row means %	k
Case Summary 1 ($n = 124$)	Minimal	94	.76	98	.90	99	.97	97	.88
Case Summary 2 ($n = 124$)	Minimal	98	.94	98	.90	98	.93	98	.92
Mock Evaluation ($n = 124$)	Moderate	66	.10	78	.31	84	.47	76	.29
Record Review ($n = 313$)	Substantial	49	.00	62	.05	84	.46	65	.17
Column Means		77	.45	84	.54	91	.71		

Note: Four different case scenarios were used. The cases in case summary 1 and mock evaluation exercises represented valid cases. The cases in case summary 2 and record review exercises represented an invalid and a highly ambiguous case, respectively.

near-adequate reliability was achieved in 2 others (i.e., mock evaluation and record review cases using NJP scoring).
2. Of the three design features tested, the degree of case ambiguity had the greatest impact on reliability. This was evident from an examination of the variation in kappas among the row means. Agreement between professionals was high when the case facts supported a single hypothesis as in case summary 1 involving a "highly probable" CSA allegation and in case summary 2 involving a "highly improbable" CSA allegation. Agreement was quite limited when the case facts nearly equally supported more than one hypothesis about the allegation's validity as in the record review exercise.
3. An examination of column means revealed that the more inclusive credible evidence standard for determining substantiations resulted in higher levels of agreement than the narrower preponderance of evidence standard, with kappa means of .54 and .45, respectively.
4. A comparison of column means suggested that excluding NJP/indeterminate cases from the agreement/disagreement tallies resulted in improved reliability, although a comparison of individual cases suggested that this improvement was not consistent across all cases.
5. In summary, these findings demonstrate that the magnitude of reliability estimates in forensic decision making studies is dependent on design features such as: (a) the degree of case ambiguity, (b) the use of a broad or narrow definition of "substantiated," and (c) exclusion or inclusion of no judgment possible/undecided cases.

These results suggest that empirical estimates of reliability are in large part an artifact of arbitrary variations of research. Consequently, until the advent of studies that (a) are ecologically valid and (b) assess agreement using representative samples of actual forensic cases, we believe caution is warranted in generalizing from research to practice.

UNSETTLED OR UNSETTLING SCIENCE?

As we have seen, analysis of the reliability and accuracy of professional judgments in CSA assessments has focused primarily on seven studies, most of which were published almost 20 years ago. Herman (2009) argues that the logical conclusion from these studies is unavoidable: forensic CSA decisions made in the absence of definitive, corroborative evidence are fundamentally and irredeemably unreliable. We have made the case that the issue is empirically far from settled. First, the studies Herman relies on are unrepresentative of actual forensic practice, and their findings cannot be generalized to the real world. Second, we describe six design features in substantiation studies that shape the reliability findings obtained. Third, we demonstrate that one can attain adequate to excellent agreement in reliability research, even using soft, psychosocial evidence, by selectively implementing one or more of the design features described.

This debate is more than an academic exercise. Herman not only condemns current child protective services and forensic practice as methodologically invalid and unethical but also recommends "reforms" that we believe would undermine the child protection efforts that have been established over the past 25 years. Among the more concerning reforms advocated is an end to "the process of making inferences about the validity of abuse allegations on the basis of psychosocial evidence, including *children's reports in investigative interviews*" (p. 258, emphasis added). This position contravenes decades of accepted CPS and forensic practice. For example, as part of a comprehensive literature review, Faller (2007) identified 16 sets of guidelines published since 1982 for determining the likely validity of CSA allegations. All 16 sets of guidelines emphasized an analysis of the child's disclosure statement as central to decision making.

However, according to our understanding of the "reform" position, one disclosure is as good as another. There is nothing to be gained by an assessment of the plausibility, consistency, or the presence of idiosyncratic or contextual details in the child's account of abuse. The child's account of alleged abuse is useful only for identifying the possible existence of definitive, corroborative evidence, not as evidence in its own right. In other words, unless the child identifies the location of the perpetrator's collection of DVDs of his or her abuse or reveals the existence of a semen-stained pair of panties, the details of his or her disclosure are viewed as irrelevant to the investigative process. The five-year-old's description of "sticky stuff like snot squirting out" of her uncle's penis when he made her "squeeze it until it gets big" adds nothing to case determination. The case remains an uncorroborated allegation of a young child versus the vigorous and compelling denials of the alleged offender. It is noteworthy that the "reform" position makes little distinction between the differing roles and differing evidence requirements for child protective services versus the criminal judicial system. In both cases, subjective assessments of the child's account of abuse are viewed as ill-advised because they involve substantial risk of false accusations of CSA against innocent adults (refer to Lyon, Ahern, & Scurich, this issue, for a further critique of Herman's views on the diagnostic utility of the child's disclosure statement).

Identifying and protecting child victims of sexual molestation and exploitation is a laudable societal value. The CPS system, together with law enforcement and the judicial system, attempt to balance the protection of children from CSA and the protection of innocent adults from false accusations, with the goal of minimizing false negative errors and false positive errors. In the service of minimizing false positive errors, the proposed "reforms" would likely severely limit the number of sexual abuse victims identified and protected. With the child's disclosure statement invalidated and other "soft" or psychosocial evidence dismissed as irrelevant, both CPS substantiations and criminal prosecution of sexual perpetrators would become extremely difficult. If definitive evidence is required to substantiate a CSA allegation, a sexual perpetrator who is careful not to cause significant physical injury to the child or to leave DNA evidence and who refrains from making a videotaped record of his or her deviant activities would likely be able to sexually exploit children with virtual impunity.

Hard, corroborative evidence is no panacea. Defense attorneys work overtime to keep such evidence out of court, with frequent success. The identity of the perpetrator or the child may be indiscernible on videos taken of the abuse. Offender confessions can be attacked as manipulated or coerced. Diagnostic medical evidence may become less definitive over time, and an opposing medical expert can almost always be found to dispute the interpretation of the findings.

In conclusion, we can all agree that erroneous decisions in forensic evaluations of alleged CSA have the potential to devastate lives. As the current discussion has revealed, however, there is no consensus on the nature and frequency of such errors and, consequently, no agreement on their method of prevention. Herman (2005, 2009) represents an extremely negative position in the debate. The remedies he proposes are radical and ill-conceived, especially given the fact that the extent of the problem of evaluator error is still unknown. Clearly, more and better research is needed, both to guide practice and to inform debate.

REFERENCES

American Professional Society on the Abuse of Children. (1997). *Guidelines for psychosocial evaluation of suspected sexual abuse in children* (2nd ed.). Elmhurst, IL: Author.

Everson, M. D. & Sandoval, J. M. (2011). Forensic child sexual abuse evaluations: Assessing subjectivity and bias in professional judgments. *Child Abuse and Neglect, 35*, 287–298.

Faller, K. C. (2007). *Interviewing children about sexual abuse: Controversies and best practice.* New York: Oxford.

Finlayson, L. M. & Koocher, G. P. (1991). Professional judgment and child abuse reporting in sexual abuse cases. *Professional Psychology: Research and Practice, 22*, 464–472.

Fleiss, J. L. (1981). *Statistical methods for rates and proportions.* New York: John Wiley & Sons.

Herman, S. (2005). Improving decision making in forensic child sexual abuse evaluations. *Law and Human Behavior, 29*(1), 87–120.

Herman, S. (2009). Forensic child sexual abuse evaluations: Accuracy, ethics and admissibility. In K. Kuehnle & M. Connell (Eds.), *The evaluation of child sexual abuse allegations: A comprehensive guide to assessment and testimony* pp. 247–266. Hoboken, NJ: Wiley.

Hershkowitz, I., Fisher, S., Lamb, M. E., & Horowitz, D. (2007). Improving credibility assessment in child sexual abuse allegations: The role of the NICHD investigative interview protocol. *Child Abuse and Neglect, 31*(2), 99–110.

Horner, T. M., Guyer, M. J., & Kalter, N. M. (1992). Prediction, prevention, and clinical expertise in child custody cases in which allegations of child sexual abuse have been made: Pt. III. Studies of expert opinion formation. *Family Law Quarterly, 26*(2), 141–170.

Horner, T. M., Guyer, M. J., & Kalter, N. M. (1993). Clinical expertise and the assessment of child sexual abuse. *Journal of the American Academy of Child and Adolescent Psychiatry, 32*(5), 925–931.

Jackson, H. & Nuttall, R. (1993). Clinician responses to sexual abuse allegations. *Child Abuse and Neglect, 17*, 127–143.

Kuehnle, K. (1996). *Assessing allegations of child sexual abuse*. Sarasota, FL: Professional Resource Press.

Kuehnle, K. (1998). Child sexual evaluations: The scientist-practioner model. *Behavioral Sciences & the Law, 16*(1), 5-20.

Kuehnle, K., & Connell, M. (2009). *The evaluation of child sexual abuse allegations: A comprehensive guide to assessment and testimony*. Hoboken, NJ: John Wiley & Sons.

Landis, R., & Koch, G. (1977). The measurement of observer agreement for categorical data. *Biometrics, 33*(1), 159–174.

Levine, M. (1998). Do standards of proof affect decision making in child protective investigations? *Law and Human Behavior, 22*, 341–347.

McGraw, J. M., & Smith, H. A. (1992). Child sexual abuse allegations amidst divorce and custody proceedings. Refining the validation. *Journal of Child Sexual Abuse, 1*, 49–62.

Oates, R. K., Jones, D. P. H., Denson, A., Sirotnak, A., Gary, N., & Krugman, R. (2000). Erroneous concerns about child sexual abuse. *Child Abuse & Neglect, 24*(1), 149–157.

Parry, C. (2009). *Statewide report: Child maltreatment identification, Part 2*. Berkeley, CA: California Social Work Education Center, School of Social Work, University of California at Berkeley.

Randolph, J. J. (2008). *Online kappa calculator*. Retrieved from http://justus.randolph.name/kappa

Realmuto, G. M., Jensen, J., & Wescoe, S. (1990). Specificity and sensitivity of sexually anatomically correct dolls in substantiating abuse: A pilot study. *Journal of the American Academy of Child and Adolescent Psychiatry, 29*(5), 743–746.

Realmuto, G. M., & Wescoe, S. (1992). Agreement among professionals about a child's sexual abuse status: Interviews with sexually anatomically correct dolls as indicators of abuse. *Child Abuse and Neglect, 126*(5), 719–725.

Shumaker, K. R. (2000). Measured professional competence between and among different mental health disciplines when evaluating and making recommendations in cases of suspected child sexual abuse. *Dissertation Abstracts International, 60*(11), 5791B (UMI No. 9950748).

U.S. Department of Human Services. (2003). *National study of child protective services systems and reform efforts*. Washington, DC: U.S. Department of Health and Human Services.

AUTHOR NOTES

Mark D. Everson, PhD, is professor of psychiatry and director of the Program on Childhood Trauma and Maltreatment at the University of North Carolina at Chapel Hill. He has served on the National Board of Directors of the American Professional Society on the Abuse of Children, and he co-chaired APSAC task forces that developed practice guidelines on investigative interviewing and on the use of anatomical dolls in cases of alleged child abuse. Dr. Everson's professional career has had a primary focus on improving forensic assessments of alleged child sexual abuse.

José Miguel Sandoval, MSc, MPhil, is a guest lecturer in statistics at the Duke University Center for International Development. Formerly he served as a statistician at the University of North Carolina Injury Prevention Research Center and at the Duke University Center on Child and Family Policy.

Nancy Berson, LCSW, is assistant director of the Program on Childhood Trauma and Maltreatment at the University of North Carolina at Chapel Hill. She has had more than 30 years of experience in working with abused and neglected children, including coordinating the Duke University Child Protection Team and working with the Guardian ad Litem Program and Departments of Social Services.

Mary Crowson, PhD, provides psychological services to maltreated children and their caregivers. Her clinical work at the University of North Carolina includes interventions for very young children who have been maltreated, psychological evaluations of children with histories of maltreatment, and expert testimony and consultation regarding child abuse disclosures and the impact of abuse.

Harriet Robinson, MSW, LCSW, currently serves as case manager in the University of North Carolina Hospital's Emergency Medicine Department. Formerly she provided clinical and forensic services at the University of North Carolina Program on Childhood Trauma and Maltreatment.

Mental Health Professionals in Children's Advocacy Centers: Is There Role Conflict?

THEODORE P. CROSS
University of Illinois at Urbana-Champaign, Urbana, Illinois, USA

JANET E. FINE
Massachusetts Office for Victim Assistance, Boston, Massachusetts, USA

LISA M. JONES and WENDY A. WALSH
University of New Hampshire, Durham, New Hampshire, USA

Two recent chapters in professional books have criticized children's advocacy centers for creating role conflict for mental health professionals because of their work with criminal justice and child protection professionals in children's advocacy centers as part of a coordinated response to child abuse. This article argues that these critiques misunderstand children's advocacy center practice and overestimate the risk of role conflict. Children's advocacy center standards set a boundary between forensic interviewing and therapy, which in most children's advocacy centers are done by separate professionals and never by the same professional for a given child. Many mental health professionals serve children's advocacy centers as consultants with no treatment role. Children's advocacy center therapists are rarely involved in investigation, and their participation in multidisciplinary teams focuses on children's interests and well-being.

Children's advocacy centers (CACs) are specialized programs designed to provide the most effective professional response to reports of child sexual abuse or other serious child abuse. More than 700 CACs have been established across the United States, with at least one in each state (according to the National Children's Alliance website [http://www.nationalchildrensalliance.org/index.php]), and 45 out of the 50 largest American cities have CACs as of this writing (Cross, 2010). CACs provide comprehensive investigation and intervention services for thousands of children every year. Coordinating criminal justice, mental health, child welfare, medical, victim advocacy, and other professionals is perhaps the most important function of CACs. It demands careful attention to establishing both appropriate linkages and appropriate boundaries among different disciplines. Recent publications have criticized CACs for creating "role conflict" for mental health professionals because of their work with criminal justice and child protection professionals in CACs (Connell, 2008; Melton & Kimbrough-Melton, 2006). Mental health professionals include professionals with a range of different training, including licensed clinical social workers, psychologists, psychiatrists, psychiatric nurses, and licensed mental health counselors. This article examines CAC practice and assesses the risk of role conflict for mental health professionals. It argues that Connell's and Melton and Kimbrough-Melton's critiques misunderstand current CAC practice and overestimate the risk of role conflict for mental health professionals in CACs.

Several sources of information were used for this article. In part, it is based on the authors' professional experiences with CACs. Cross, Jones, and Walsh have conducted a multisite evaluation of CACs (see e.g., Cross et al., 2008). Fine has been a director of two CACs, has previously served on the Standards Committee of the National Children's Alliance (NCA), the membership organization of CACs, and currently serves on the NCA Board of Directors. Fine and Cross also serve on the board of directors of a state chapter of the NCA. In addition, the current NCA standards governing CAC practice were reviewed (see National Children's Alliance, 2008) as was a CAC directors' manual on mental health services (Child Welfare Committee, National Child Traumatic Stress Network, & National Children's Alliance 2008) that was developed by a joint committee of the NCA and the National Child Traumatic Stress Network, an organization devoted to improving care for traumatized children. Finally, we interviewed the executive director of the NCA and three current or former CAC directors involved in writing the current NCA standards. These key informants were provided copies of the Melton and Kimbrough-Melton and Connell articles to review and were queried about the potential for role conflict of mental health professionals in current CAC practice.

CONCERNS ABOUT ROLE CONFLICT

The Melton and Kimbrough-Melton (2006) and Connell (2008) publications expressing concerns about role conflict for mental health professionals in CACs are both chapters in professional books in fields relevant to child sexual abuse. These authors argue that mental health professionals involved in CACs serve in multiple roles, both providing children with mental health treatment and also serving as (a) forensic evaluators of reports of abuse and (b) collaborators with criminal justice and child protection professionals on gathering evidence for court actions. These latter roles conflict with their role as treatment providers. The court actions referred to include criminal prosecution of child abuse and civil court actions regarding child placement, custody, visitation, and other decisions about the child. Melton and Kimbrough-Melton and Connell argue that these role conflicts interfere with mental health professionals' responsibility to provide effective and ethical mental health services.

Melton and Kimbrough-Melton explain their concern about role conflict as follows:

> Because of their presumed skill in interviewing children, the mental health professionals may conduct many or all of the investigatory interviews on which CPS [child protective services], police and prosecutors rely. Even when mental health professionals in such settings do not themselves conduct the investigatory interviews, they are likely to participate as team members in prosecutorial decision-making, and information that they gather in therapeutic interviews may be used in the team process. Thus, clinicians directly or indirectly participate in the gathering of evidence to determine, among other possible decisions, whether child maltreatment has occurred, a dependency petition will be filed in family court, criminal or juvenile charges will be brought against a suspect, the child will be placed into an emergency shelter or foster care, restrictions will be placed on the child's contact with parents, or both. Besides often acting directly as therapists and advocates to help alleviate a crisis, mental health professionals become actively engaged as prosecutorial investigators and decision makers. (p. 36)

Melton and Kimbrough-Melton express concern about two different possible consequences of the role conflict they describe:

> First, if a mental health professional becomes concerned with gathering evidence and helping the prosecution to make its case (whether for conviction and incarceration of an incestuous father or civil adjudication of abuse, placement of the child in foster care, and ultimately termination of parental rights), will the clinician's ability to function as a therapist for the child or the family be compromised? Indeed, will the slippage into law enforcement activities compromise that clinician's ability—or even

other clinicians' ability—to help other children and families? Second, will adoption of an explicit stance of children's advocate compromise mental health professionals' ability to act as unbiased experts? (p. 37)

Melton and Kimbrough-Melton's concerns are not just about the involvement of the mental health professional in the CAC's multidisciplinary team but also about their employment in an organization affiliated with the prosecutor:

> Although these multiple roles (or a subset of them) can arise no matter what the auspice for the clinician's work, employment in a prosecution-affiliated facility makes the potential role conflicts explicit. Even if investigatory staff are physically separated from therapeutic staff as mentioned by Congressman Cramer, the problems persist of (a) possible spillover effects from proximity and contact with investigative staff on perceptions of clinicians among clients and the general public and (b) at least the appearance of bias in clinicians' judgments. The former possible effects can impede the clinicians' ability to act as effective therapists; the latter can affect adversely their objectivity as experts and clinical evaluators. (p. 37)

The other chapter that expresses concern about role conflict of mental health professionals in CACs is Connell's (2008) chapter on children's advocacy centers in a guidebook on evaluation of sexual allegations. Connell (p. 436) quotes Faller and Palusci (2007, p. 1027), who say that "more success in prosecution" is "a primary goal of the CAC movement." Connell then warns about conflict between mental health professionals' need to be neutral and objective regarding the question of alleged abuse and CACs' interest in prosecution:

> Truth-seeking, prosecuting, protecting and treating, then, are in some ways incompatible undertakings. In an environment charged with protecting children by increasing prosecutions, there may be an inherent bias toward perceiving children as victims or as suspected victims of sexual abuse. If this bias exists, a child who has not been abused may be caught in a situation where denial of abuse is less likely to be believed. (p. 439)

Connell also cites Melton and Kimbrough-Melton (2006) to argue for the risk of role conflict and gives the issue of role conflict a prominent place in her conclusion section. Connell writes:

> The overarching concern with the CAC model is the fundamental problems of diverse goals of the disciplines represented in the CAC effort. As Melton and Kimbrough-Melton (2006) noted, there may be inherent

problems in combining advocacy efforts with truth-seeking, particularly when successful advocacy is measured by increased prosecutions. (p. 443)

In a boxed set of bullet points titled "Guidelines" at the end of the chapter, Connell is less tentative: "There are inherent role conflicts of the multidisciplinary team approach" (p. 445).

In her chapter, Connell also expresses concern about extended forensic evaluation, a model employed in less than 10% of CACs in which children who do not disclose abuse to investigators but exhibit behaviors that are strongly suggestive of victimization and/or trauma are referred for specialized multisession evaluations. In addition, she raises questions about maintenance of official records of forensic interviews in CACs. Connell's other concerns are beyond the scope of this article.

HOW CACs WORK

To consider the risk of role conflict in CACs, it is important to understand concretely how CACs work and how different professionals actually participate in them. CACs are usually independent, nonprofit organizations, but sometimes are a program of a prosecutor's office, hospital, or other nonprofit agency. They are required to be housed in a dedicated, child-friendly setting and designed to be physically and psychologically safe for clients.

To be an accredited CAC, a center must follow a set of practice standards developed by the National Children's Alliance. Accreditation is not only prized as an indication of professional competence and quality but is also tied to the distribution of federal dollars to CACs through state NCA chapters. The first set of accreditation standards took effect in 2000 and an updated set were developed in 2008 and took effect January 2010. The standards address the following 10 areas: multidisciplinary team, cultural competency and diversity, forensic interviews, victim support and advocacy, medical evaluation, mental health, case review, case tracking, organizational capacity, and child-focused setting.

The following seven types of professionals at a minimum participate in a CAC: law enforcement, child protection, prosecution, medical health, mental health, victim advocacy, and CAC (i.e., a dedicated staff member of the CAC). Other professionals beyond this core group may also be involved. Professionals who collaborate with the CAC are usually employed by and accountable to their primary agencies, although some participate as private practitioners. Each professional does his or her specific job but also shares information and coordinates activities as appropriate with other professionals in the CAC.

Multidisciplinary Teams

The central mechanism for coordinating professionals is the multidisciplinary team (MDT), which the NCA standards describe as the "foundation" of a CAC. Through MDTs, the CAC coordinates the efforts of multiple professionals from the first report of the case to the center to case closing. This coordination is designed to reduce stress to the child and family by eliminating redundant interventions (e.g., multiple investigative interviews by multiple professionals) and providing greater coherence and a focal point of contact for the family while allowing each agency and professional to pursue its own mission. The MDT aims to foster improved communication among agencies and facilitates the sharing of important information. In addition, the MDT is thought to enhance the quality of decision making because multiple professionals with different expertise and knowledge learn from one another and help clients receive critical information and services. Individual MDT members and their parent agencies are ultimately responsible for their own decisions; the MDT simply provides a method for making informed decisions.

There is considerable ambiguity about the term *multidisciplinary team*. The term does not refer to a fixed group of people or committee but instead to a general, multidisciplinary approach to addressing a variety of needs that arise within and across cases over time. The specific professionals involved in a MDT will vary from case to case depending on what agencies are involved and who is assigned the case; moreover, which professionals make up the MDT for a given case can change over time depending on the needs of a case. The number of individuals who participate in MDTs across cases can be substantial, if, for example, the CAC serves an area with 10 different police agencies, three different CPS offices, and four hospitals or clinics that serve child victims. Smaller jurisdictions may have more consistent teams.

The Investigation Team

One important MDT in a CAC is the multidisciplinary investigation team, which will typically convene on the child and family's entry to the CAC. At a minimum, the investigation team includes a specialized child forensic interviewer, a police investigator, and an investigating caseworker (if CPS is involved). Sometimes the investigating officer or caseworker has the specialized training to conduct the child forensic interview and those two functions will be performed by one person. Often prosecutors, victim witness advocates, and medical professionals will participate as well. Mental health professionals may be involved at this point, as we'll discuss in more detail.

For verbal children, a key part of the investigation team's work is the child forensic interview, which is designed to elicit as much information regarding the allegations as possible in a nonleading manner to assist in providing additional direction for the criminal and child protective investigations. While the child forensic interviewer talks to the child, the multidisciplinary investigation team typically observes the interview through a one-way mirror or closed circuit television. A forensic interview typically serves the investigative needs of both law enforcement and child protective agencies and also informs the clinical assessment of the child. Following the interview, the team is responsible for coordinating a comprehensive response plan with the actual interventions being carried out by individual professionals.

The Forensic Interviewer

In many CACs, the forensic interviewer is a dedicated specialist employed by the CAC. In other CACs, forensic interviews are conducted by trained professionals of agencies with a statutory responsibility for investigation: CPS investigative caseworkers or law enforcement officers. CAC forensic interviewers must receive specialized training in reliable forensic interview techniques, child development, question typologies, and the cognitive and emotional impact of trauma (refer to Olafson, this issue, for a discussion of current practice in child forensic interviewing). The NCA standards (2008) clearly distinguish between the role of the forensic interviewer and the role of the therapist (see also, Child Welfare Committee et al., 2008). NCA standards state that "Every effort should be made to maintain clear boundaries between these roles and processes" (p. 26) and require each CAC to document in writing how the forensic process is separate from mental health treatment. Standard practice in CACs is for these two functions in a case to be carried out by different professionals. Indeed, in our experience and that of our informants, in the overwhelming majority of CACs forensic interviewers never provide treatment to CAC clients, and therapists working with CAC clients never conduct forensic interviews. In a very small number of CACs, mental health professionals conduct forensic interviews on some cases and provide treatment on others, but even then, the same professional does not perform both functions with the same child due to some of the concerns stated in the Connell and Melton and Melton-Kimbrough chapters.

While some forensic interviewers have a mental health professional background, most do not. Data from 468 professionals who were trained in forensic interviewing between February 2008 and July 2010 at the National Children's Advocacy Center in Huntsville, Alabama, one of the largest training centers in the country, show that only 9.6% identified themselves as mental health or treatment professionals (Leith, 2010). Others may have had a mental health educational background (e.g., a BSW or MSW) but identified their discipline as forensic interviewer or child protective services worker. When such professionals do have a mental health professional background, they typically fit the description of the forensic specialist that Melton and colleagues describe as pivotal in a system that maintains appropriate boundaries, that is, "mental health professionals whose work *primarily* or *solely* consists of conducting evaluations for the legal system" (Melton and Kimbrough-Melton, 2006, p. 30; see also Melton, Petrila, Poythress & Slobogin, 1997).

Case Review

CACs also conduct regular multidisciplinary team case review meetings to share information and discuss what needs to be done on a case. According to the NCA Standards (NCA, 2008), the case review process performs the following functions, depending on the needs of the case:

1. Review interview outcomes.
2. Discuss, plan, and monitor the progress of the investigation.
3. Review medical evaluations.
4. Discuss child protection and other safety issues.
5. Provide input for prosecution and sentencing decisions.
6. Discuss emotional support and treatment needs of the child and nonoffending family members and strategies for meeting those needs.
7. Assess the family's reactions and response to the child's disclosure.
8. Review criminal and civil dependency case disposition.
9. Make provisions for court education and court support.
10. Discuss cross-cultural issues relevant to the case. (p. 29)

The CAC can continue to be involved with a family regarding investigation, often intermittently, over an extended period of time, if, for example, criminal and child protection proceedings take time. CACs will often provide support to families if and when the case goes to court and the child needs to participate.

Mental Health Professionals' Involvement in CACs

Different communities make different choices about how and when mental health professionals are involved in the CAC. An important distinction is that sometimes a mental health professional is involved in a multidisciplinary team because he or she is the therapist of a child served by a CAC, and sometimes a mental health professional serves purely as a consultant, with no therapeutic relationships with CAC clients.

Therapists are not involved in the initial investigation team. A few CACs involve mental health consultants in the investigation team, but most CACs do not have this resource. A mental health consultant's expertise in such areas as child development and trauma response may help a forensic interviewer frame questions to the child in the interview or help the team understand the child's responses; they can also help assess the mental health needs of family members and assist with referrals.

Mental health professionals are more frequently involved in CAC multidisciplinary teams during case review. Because case review meetings usually consider multiple cases, the mental health professional is typically a consultant. However, given signed consent from the child's legal guardian, a therapist may attend for that portion of the meeting in which the team discusses the child the therapist is treating. Some CACs have linkage agreements with clinics or private practitioners who are external to the CAC but who participate in multidisciplinary teams. Other CACs employ therapists who provide mental health treatment to children at the center.

Involvement of the mental health consultant and/or the child's therapist in multidisciplinary team can legitimately advance children's best interests (Child Welfare Committee et al., 2008). Mental health professionals are often the best qualified to advise other team members about the emotional impact of their actions on children and families. Mental health consultants can also help team members take into account children's level of development when interpreting children's behavior and when communicating with them. Therapists' involvement is likely to be limited to confirming that the child is involved in therapy, communicating the child and family's concerns related to the response of other agencies, and, like the consultants, suggesting steps to prevent further harm to the child. Therapists can also learn about next steps that prosecutors, child protection agencies, and others are planning to take and thereby can better help families cope with these actions.

Mental health professionals may be called on to testify in criminal or civil court, but this would not be a function of their involvement in the MDT or CAC, although that may make prosecutors more knowledgeable about them. They may testify as expert witnesses about such matters as the behavioral effects of abuse. The law is likely to prevent them from talking about what the child says in treatment or assessment (hearsay evidence), and it certainly will not allow them to speak to the ultimate issue of whether or not abuse occurred, which is a matter for the judge or jury to decide. There is more flexibility about what mental health professionals can say in child protection cases, although even here they are enjoined from speaking about the ultimate issue. Mental health professionals perform this function in court because of their expertise, with or without MDTs and CACs.

ANALYSIS OF CONCERNS ABOUT ROLE CONFLICT

The review of CAC practice above provides a basis for analyzing the concerns about role conflict expressed by Melton and Kimbrough-Melton (2006) and Connell (2008). Below we examine these authors' arguments in light of current knowledge of CAC practice.

Mental Health Professionals as Forensic Interviewers

Melton and Kimbrough-Melton (2006) state that "mental health professionals may conduct many or all of the investigatory interviews on which CPS, police and prosecutors rely" (p. 36). However, the available data show that this is rarely true. Leith's (2010) training data suggest that only a small percentage of professionals engaged in forensic interviewer training are mental health professionals. And even when mental health professionals *do* conduct forensic interviews, role conflict is not a concern because they are not functioning as treatment providers. In line with the NCA Standards requiring a clear boundary between conducting forensic interviews and providing treatment, CACs have separated these two functions. In the vast majority of CACs, these functions are provided by dedicated specialists who do not perform the other function.

In a small number of CACs, there are mental health professionals who do forensic interviews with some children and provide therapy to others. About this circumstance, Melton and Kimbrough-Melton express concern about a "slippage into law enforcement activities" (p. 37) that will compromise the therapist's capacity to help *other* children and families. This sounds plausible, but it is also plausible that reasonably well-trained professionals can maintain appropriate boundaries as they work with different cases. Ultimately this is an empirical question. Its relevance for making judgments about CACs is limited, however, given the infrequency with which any mental health professionals conduct forensic interviews and also provide treatment to children in a CAC.

Mental Health Professionals as Prosecutorial Investigators

Melton and Kimbrough-Melton express concern that, through their participation in CACs, mental health professionals will be influenced to assist investigation, prosecution, and other court-related actions in a way that will conflict with their primary mission. There are several grounds on which to question Melton and Kimbrough-Melton's argument. First, their text seems to convey the assumption that mental health professionals involved in a CAC/MDT response to a child would necessarily have a treatment relationship with that child. They use the terms *mental health professional*, *clinician*, and *therapist* interchangeably and ask "will the clinician's ability to function as a therapist for the child or the family be compromised?" (p. 37). As discussed above, however, mental health professionals often participate in MDTs as consultants without serving as clinicians. These professionals are unlikely even to have direct contact with children and families. Because the child's best interest is the primary principle guiding the MDT, the mental health consultant will make recommendations to promote the child's well-being but can also help investigators without any possibility of role conflict because they do not have a treatment relationship with the child and family.

Second, even when the child's therapist participates in the MDT, the involvement is limited and the chances of a role conflict are therefore less than Melton and Kimbrough-Melton suggest. Children's therapists rarely, if ever, participate in the investigation team, which typically includes only professionals with dedicated investigation responsibilities. When therapists participate in case reviews, it often is for a limited period of time, and their focus is on the child's well-being and not on the investigation. Most prosecutors keep some distance between prosecution and children's therapy, both to protect children's privacy and to avoid defense attorneys obtaining information from the therapy through discovery and using it to raise questions about children's credibility.

Third, in some circumstances, therapists' assistance to criminal justice and child protection professionals is *not* role conflict but instead good practice in children's interest. Their perception that justice has been done is important to child victims (see Melton, 1992: Melton & Limber, 1989), and child victims and nonoffending caregivers often have an interest in prosecuting offenders, which can help children feel safer and support their credibility. Good therapists are not removed from the legal process but instead explore with children and families the purposes and potential outcomes of legal intervention and help them weigh the pros and cons of participating in the criminal justice system. As Melton and Limber (1989) recommend, "the general strategy should be to make children partners in the pursuit of justice" (p. 1227). Therapists can also assist children and families in better understanding various goals of participating in the system in addition to, or instead of, a criminal conviction. This may or may not comport with the prosecution's goals. Child victims and families may similarly favor certain child protective interventions, and therapists can also play a role in assisting families in decision-making related to these.

If therapists have assessed children's and caregivers' wishes and their interests accurately and secured children's assent and nonoffending caregivers' informed consent, there are circumstances in which it is appropriate for therapists to join with the family to assist prosecution and child protection professionals. It would be misleading and an overstatement to describe this as being "actively engaged as prosecutorial investigators" (Melton & Kimbrough-Melton, 2006, p. 36) since it mostly involves either appropriately sharing information or supporting children and families in the legal process. With the child and family's consent and support, therapists may be able to share information from the treatment that would assist investigation or prosecution, such as observations of child behavior that might reflect the impact of abuse. Therapists may also be able to assist both children and prosecutors appropriately if cases go to trial. For example, therapists may advise prosecutors about when children may be emotionally ready to testify and may suggest strategies to help prepare a child for the courtroom experience. They may serve as an extra support person in court for the child and, at sentencing, may work with victim witness advocates and the child to prepare a developmentally appropriate victim impact statement.

Truth-Seeking and Prosecution

Connell suggests that "truth-seeking" and "prosecuting" are "in some ways incompatible undertakings." By this she implies that truth-seeking is secondary for prosecutors filing criminal charges. The suggested dichotomy is false. Indeed, Connell impugns prosecutors by suggesting that prosecuting and truth-seeking are incompatible. The CAC investigation method assumes that the accuracy of the allegation is unknown at the outset. This is a principle that is critical to criminal prosecution given the high standard of proof and the ensuing potential consequences (loss of liberty) for those accused. Truth-seeking serves the goal of successful prosecution and is not undermined by it.

Connell's concern may to some degree reflect misunderstanding of current prosecution practice in CACs. CACs are not as prosecution-oriented as the two chapters might suggest. Melton and Kimbrough-Melton focus on the National Children's Advocacy Center, the first CAC and one that was formed under the leadership of the district attorney. However, most CACs are independent, nonprofit organizations, and many are hospital-based or part of larger nonprofits. Only a minority of CACs are based in prosecutor offices.

While former District Attorney Robert "Bud" Cramer is considered the "father" of the CAC model, criminal prosecution was never considered the overriding goal of the multidisciplinary team model. Connell cites Faller and Palusci (2007) on successful prosecution as "a primary goal of the CAC movement" (Connell, 2009, p. 436), but it is not *the* primary goal, nor is it likely that Faller and Palusci meant to suggest that prosecution was such an important goal that it supersedes the need to seek the truth. While offender accountability has been an increasing focus in child abuse cases over the past three decades, both in and out of CACs, it is not the driving force behind most CAC interventions regardless of CAC sponsorship or venue. Research suggests that CACs vary considerably in the importance they place on prosecution and the range of cases they think should be prosecuted (Walsh, Jones, & Cross, 2003). In any CAC, prosecution is a fairly uncommon intervention. Connell (2008) cites NCA data that 10% of cases are accepted for prosecution, which is consistent with a meta-analysis that shows that only a minority of cases referred to district attorneys' offices are prosecuted (Cross, Walsh, Simone, & Jones, 2003). In fact, in the majority of cases in which prosecution does not ensue, the prosecutor assumes an inactive role on the team while those responsible for protective and treatment services coordinate for the duration of that individual case. References to a prosecution versus a therapeutic model are contrary to the core concepts of a CAC—it is not *either/or* but *both/and*. Apart from prosecution, most CACs measure themselves as much if not more by the delivery and effectiveness of child protection, victim advocacy, and treatment services, along with the degree to which victims and their nonoffending family members are afforded their rights and participate meaningfully in the process.

Inherent Role Conflict

Connell's statement that "there are inherent role conflicts of the multidisciplinary team approach" (p. 445) needs close analysis. If a role conflict is "inherent" to the multidisciplinary team approach, then this might cast doubt on the use of multidisciplinary teams altogether, and any professional who participates in an MDT would wittingly or unwittingly compromise his or her professional integrity. Connell and Melton and Kimbrough-Melton do not really discuss the process through which involvement in the multidisciplinary team meeting is supposed to lead to role conflict. Presumably therapists' interactions with criminal justice and child protection professionals influences them to a degree that overwhelms their attention to their ethical responsibilities. Even if such influence-through-interaction occurs, is it actually more likely to happen in a multidisciplinary team? There is a sparse research literature on professionals in multidisciplinary child abuse teams, and it is not very helpful on this question. Studies like those of Kolbo and Strong (1997) and Jensen, Jacobson, Unrau, and Robinson (1996) found that professionals reported satisfaction with their experiences in multidisciplinary teams but lack data on professional behavior. Bell (2001) found that prosecution staff participated significantly more than other professionals in MDTs in 15 multidisciplinary child protection teams in New Jersey and that mental health staff were among the professionals who participated least, but there were no data on effect on mental health staff's behavior or decision making.

Therapists could circumvent the possibility of influence by other professionals by avoiding all contact with criminal justice and child protection professionals, but such contact may be necessary for the child's treatment (e.g., when the therapist needs to know what the child will be asked to do in court), and such avoidance would do a disservice to the child. Clearly therapists are sometimes obliged to talk to police and CPS. When they do, role conflict is also possible when therapists are solo professionals or working in agencies with little connection with prosecution and child protection agencies. Indeed, therapists working in well-functioning multidisciplinary teams may be in a better position to avoid role conflict. The group process in the MDT can develop an overarching attention to the best interests of the child that supersedes any one agency's agenda. The MDT has developed protocols with input from all disciplines that reflect the responsibilities and ethical principles of all team members and govern communication and decision making. Full involvement of all the disciplines may allow for each professional on the MDT to focus more comfortably on his/her own specific function. Individual members of the team could be supported by the group against any effort by one team member to dominate. Agencies involved in MDTs may have greater experience dealing with other disciplines. Clearly there is nothing intrinsic in how a multidisciplinary team works nor any data that suggest that role conflict would be *inherent* in a multidisciplinary team.

Employment in a Prosecution-Affiliated Facility

Melton and Kimbrough-Melton express concern about "spillover effects from proximity and contact with investigative staff on perceptions of clinicians among clients and the general public" (p. 37) when therapists work in a CAC that is a "prosecution-affiliated facility" (p. 37). They cite the example of the National Children's Advocacy Center (NCAC) in Huntsville, Alabama, that has a separate small set of therapy offices as part of the CAC. There are several factors, however, that should reduce concern about spillover effects. First, the actual proximity of and contact between therapists and investigative staff in CACs is generally more circumscribed than the NCAC example might suggest. In the vast majority of CACs, criminal justice and mental health staff work in different locations. Most CACs are *not* based in investigative agencies, and most do *not* have mental health professionals on staff. Those CACs that are based in prosecutors' offices are particularly unlikely to have therapists on staff, both because these agencies are neither skilled nor invested in providing treatment services and because many are interested in maintaining some distance from treatment professionals, as discussed above.

Second, even when there is proximity and contact between therapeutic and investigative staff, such as when CACs provide on-site mental health services, it seems unlikely that it would affect "perceptions of clinicians among clients and the general public" in the vast majority of cases. In many cases, as we have discussed above, child victims and nonoffending caregivers will have an interest in pursuing investigations and will perceive no conflict in an agency that houses both trauma-related mental health services and investigation functions. In fact, locating therapeutic services in CACs and thereby making them available and logistically and financially accessible may increase the number of child victims who receive treatment. Second, most of the public has little or no knowledge about CACs. The vast majority of referrals to CACs come from child protective, law enforcement, and health organizations. While CACs respond with empathy and assistance if families call, the CAC is usually a second-line responder. To the extent that members of the public know about CACs, they typically have a global view of CACs as centers that help child victims, and they endorse in general the goals of effective treatment and investigation. Members of the public who know about CACs probably have limited understanding of the participants in an

MDT and the interaction among them. Given this reality, it seems unlikely that the proximity and contact between therapeutic and investigative staff will have much of an effect on public perception of therapists working in CACs.

Melton and Kimbrough-Melton also express concern that employment in a prosecution-affiliated facility would impair mental health professionals' "objectivity as experts and clinical evaluators" (p. 37). As we have noted above, forensic interviewers are rarely mental health professionals, and a child's therapist does not conduct the forensic interview for that child. But let us consider any situation in which a mental health professional working in a CAC, therapist or not, applies his or her expertise and clinical judgment on behalf of a child. Could his or her objectivity be impaired by employment in a prosecution-affiliated facility? This is only plausible if we assume that prosecutors are at special risk for losing objectivity and then influence their CAC colleagues in other disciplines to stray from objectivity as well. This is unlikely.

NEED FOR RESEARCH

One of the difficulties of assessing Connell's and Melton and Kimbrough-Melton's claims about role conflict is that empirical data are not available about how CACs are structured and how professionals function within them. As Connell's (2008) review makes clear, research on CACs has been limited. Ultimately the degree of risk of role conflict in CACs is an empirical question, and we agree with Connell (2008) that studies are needed in this area. Surveys of CACs could be conducted to produce descriptive statistics on how mental health professionals participate in MDTs and other CAC functions and specifically how CACs maintain clear boundaries between the roles of forensic interviewer and therapist. Semistructured interviews could be conducted with samples of mental health professionals in CACs to explore how they manage practice in CACs and in what ways they communicate and collaborate with other disciplines. Observational methods could examine patterns of interaction in team meetings. One component of survey or interview studies might be to solicit examples of cases or events in which role conflict occurred or there was a risk of role conflict and study the resulting sample of case examples.

CONCLUSION

In summary, a review of how CACs work suggests that Melton and Kimbrough-Melton (2006) and Connell (2008) overestimate the risk of role conflict for mental health professionals working in CACs. CAC standards set a boundary between forensic interviewing and providing therapy, functions that are never conducted by the same professional for a given child and in most CACs are conducted by separate sets of professionals. Few forensic interviewers are mental health professionals or provide treatment services. Many mental health professionals in CACs are consultants and do not risk role conflict because they do not treat children through the CAC. Child therapists are rarely involved in the investigation, and their participation in MDTs is typically focused on children's interests and well-being. Truth-seeking serves the goal of successful prosecution and is not incompatible with it. There are no data to suggest that role conflict is inherent for multi-disciplinary teams. CACs are not as prosecution-oriented as the two chapters might suggest, since only small percentages of cases are prosecuted, and most CACs measure themselves as much if not more by service delivery and promoting victims' rights and participation than by prosecuting or obtaining convictions. Substantial concern about real or apparent role conflict for mental health professionals employed at prosecution-affiliated facilities is not warranted, because contact between prosecutors and therapists is circumscribed, prosecutors share an investment in objectivity, and the public is unlikely to consider therapist involvement as role conflict.

Although we argue that a number of factors mitigate the risk, it is impossible to rule out altogether the possibility of role conflict for mental health professionals in CACs. The National Children's Alliance has and should continue to identify specific CAC practice situations in which mental health professionals might be at risk for role conflict and offer strategies for avoiding or appropriately addressing such conflicts. In some situations, therapists, or law enforcement professionals for that matter, may need to recuse themselves from participating in certain meetings or from portions of certain meetings. While we cannot account for all current MDT and CAC practices throughout the country, the importance of clear boundaries between forensic interviewing and therapeutic intervention is central to the CAC model. It is codified in national accreditation standards and reinforced through training and dissemination of best practices by NCA and its affiliates. Given all the potential benefits of the involvement of mental health professionals in children's advocacy centers, undue concern about role conflict, which might lead to decreased participation of mental health professionals in CACs, could work against the best interests of children.

REFERENCES

Bell, L. (2001). Patterns of interaction in multidisciplinary child protection teams in New Jersey. *Child Abuse & Neglect, 25*, 65–80.

Child Welfare Committee, National Child Traumatic Stress Network, & National Children's Alliance. (2008). *CAC directors' guide to mental health services for abused children.* Los Angeles: National Center for Child Traumatic Stress.

Connell, M. (2009). The Child Advocacy Center model. In K. Kuehnle & M. Connell (Eds.), *The evaluation of child sexual allegations: A comprehensive guide to assessment and testimony* (pp. 423–449). Hoboken, NJ: John Wiley & Sons.

Cross, T. P. (2010). *Analysis of National Children's Alliance and U.S. Census data* [Unpublished raw data] Urbana, IL: University of Illinois at Urbana-Champaign.

Cross, T. P., Jones, L. J., Walsh, W., Simone, M., Kolko, D. J., Szczepanski, J., et al. (2008). The multi-site evaluation of Children's Advocacy Centers: Overview of the results and implications for practice. [Bulletin.] *OJJDP Crimes Against Children Series*. Washington, DC: Office of Juvenile Justice and Delinquency Prevention, U.S. Department of Justice.

Cross, T. P., Walsh, W., Simone, M., & Jones, L. M. (2003). Prosecution of child abuse: A meta-analysis of rates of criminal justice decisions. *Trauma, Violence and Abuse, 4*, 323–340.

Faller, K. C., & Palusci, V. J. (2007). Children's advocacy centers: Do they lead to positive case outcome? *Child Abuse & Neglect, 31*, 1021–1029.

Jensen, J. M., Jacobson, M., Unrau, Y., & Robinson, R. L. (1996). Intervention for victims of child sexual abuse: An evaluation of the children's advocacy model. *Child and Adolescent Social Work Journal, 13*, 139–156.

Kolbo, J. R., & Strong, E. (1997). Multidisciplinary team approaches to the investigation and resolution of child abuse and neglect: A national survey. *Child Maltreatment, 2*, 61–72.

Leith, A. (2010). *Analysis of 2008–2010 forensic interviewer training data* [Unpublished raw data] Huntsville, AL: National Children's Advocacy Center.

Melton, G. B. (1992). Children as partners for justice: Next steps for developmentalists. *Monographs of the Society for Research in Child Development, 57*, 153–159.

Melton, G. B., & Kimbrough-Melton, R. J. (2006). Integrating assessment, treatment and jusice: Pipe dream or possibility. In S. Sparta & G. Koocher (Eds.), *Forensic mental health assessment of children and adolescents* (pp. 30–45). New York: Oxford University Press.

Melton, G. B., & Limber, S. (1989). Psychologists' involvement in cases of child maltreatment: Limits of role and expertise. *American Psychologist, 44*, 1225–1233.

Melton, G. B., Petrila, J., Poythress, N. G., & Slobogin, C. (1997). *Psychological evaluation for the courts: A handbook for mental health professionals and lawyers* (2nd ed.). New York: Guilford.

National Children's Alliance. (2008). *Standards for accredited members* (revised 2008). Washington, DC: Author.

Walsh, W., Jones, L. M., & Cross, T. P. (2003). Children Advocacy Centers: One model, many programs. *APSAC Advisor, 15*(3), 3–7.

AUTHOR NOTES

Theodore P. Cross is a research full professor at the Children and Family Research Center in the School of Social Work at the University of Illinois at Urbana-Champaign. He directed the Multisite Evaluation of Children's

Advocacy Centers and has published numerous studies for more than 21 years on the investigation and response to child abuse.

Janet E. Fine, MS, is the executive director of the Massachusetts Office for Victim Assistance and for the past 28 years has been a leader in victim rights and services and the development of multidisciplinary teams and Children's Advocacy Centers (CAC). She was a founder of two CACs in Massachusetts and the Massachusetts Children's Alliance, chaired the committee that created the national standards for CACs, and currently serves on the National Children's Alliance Board.

Lisa M. Jones, PhD, is a research associate professor of psychology at the Crimes Against Children Research Center at the University of New Hampshire. She has been conducting research on issues of child victimization intervention and prevention for more than10 years, including research on CACs, child maltreatment trends, children's experiences with sexual abuse investigations, and Internet crimes against children.

Wendy A. Walsh, PhD, is a research associate professor of sociology at the Crimes Against Children Research Center at the University of New Hampshire. She conducts applied research on the system response to child maltreatment, including Children's Advocacy Centers, access to services for victims, and criminal justice outcomes.

Base Rates, Multiple Indicators, and Comprehensive Forensic Evaluations: Why Sexualized Behavior Still Counts in Assessments of Child Sexual Abuse Allegations

MARK D. EVERSON
University of North Carolina at Chapel Hill, Chapel Hill, North Carolina, USA

KATHLEEN COULBORN FALLER
University of Michigan, Ann Arbor, Michigan, USA

Developmentally inappropriate sexual behavior has long been viewed as a possible indicator of child sexual abuse. In recent years, however, the utility of sexualized behavior in forensic assessments of alleged child sexual abuse has been seriously challenged. This article addresses a number of the concerns that have been raised about the diagnostic value of sexualized behavior, including the claim that when population base rates for abuse are properly taken into account, the diagnostic value of sexualized behavior is insignificant. This article also identifies a best practice comprehensive evaluation model with a methodology that is effective in mitigating such concerns.

PROLOGUE

First year resident to hospital emergency room patient, a 60-year-old male clutching his chest: "I don't want to hear any more about your chest pains. Do you have any idea how many men your age come in here complaining of chest pains? Or how often chest pains are misdiagnosed as heart-related? Chest pains can be caused by a number of benign medical conditions, so the odds are that yours are nothing serious. Besides, your chest pains are what got you admitted to the ER. Statistically speaking, it would be inappropriate for us to give them any weight now in the diagnostic process. So, unless you have other symptoms to report, we'll be sending you home."

INTRODUCTION

Child forensic evaluators can readily empathize with the ER patient in the prologue. The medical resident's cavalier dismissal of the diagnostic significance of acute chest pains is analogous to recent challenges to the use of age-inappropriate sexual behavior in forensic assessments of child sexual abuse (CSA). The resident's rationale for ignoring the patient's symptoms closely parallels the reasoning used to question the diagnostic value of sexualized behavior. Additionally, the resident in this hypothetical example and many critics of current forensic practice converge in their emphasis on specificity over sensitivity in case decisions. Specificity (minimizing inclusion of false cases) and sensitivity (maximizing the inclusion of true cases) are counterbalancing indices of decision accuracy. Favoring specificity over sensitivity means that overdiagnosing CSA (a false positive error) is considered to be a more serious concern than failing to substantiate true cases of abuse (a false negative error) (Everson & Sandoval, 2011; Faller & Everson, this issue).

The purpose of this article is to address mounting concerns about the "diagnostic" value of sexualized behavior or sexual behavior problems in forensic assessments of CSA (e.g., Ceci & Bruck, 1995; Poole & Lindsay, 1998). These concerns approach their peak in book chapters by Faust, Bridges, and Ahern (2009a, 2009b); Bridges, Faust, and Ahern (2009); and Poole and Wolfe (2009) in Kuehnle and Connell's (2009) edited volume on child sexual abuse evaluations. Faust and his colleagues employ the opening three chapters of the book as a forum for condemning the field of forensic assessment for its "unwarranted" use of sexualized behavior and other behavior symptoms as possible indicators or evidence of sexual abuse. The authors cite the "unverified" and "limited" diagnostic value of such behavior indicators and the "grave" risk of false positive decision errors inherent in their use. In a fourth chapter titled "Child Development: Normative Sexual and Nonsexual Behaviors That May Be Confused With Symptoms of Sexual Abuse," Poole and Wolfe (2009) warn forensic evaluators of the risks of misinterpreting normal sexual behavior in children or sexual behavior originating from nonabuse sources, as evidence of sexual abuse. Although Poole and Wolfe as well as Faust and associates seem to dismiss the use of any behavior symptom as a possible indicator of abuse, both sets of authors single out the use of sexualized behavior in forensic decision making for specific criticism.

Our response to such criticism begins with a discussion of why aberrant and precocious sexual behavior can be an outcome of sexual abuse. Second, we examine the multiple roles that such sexual behavior problems play as abuse indicators in the forensic assessment process. Third, we identify a specific comprehensive evaluation model as an example of best practice. Fourth, we address the major concerns that Poole, Wolfe, Faust, Bridge, and Ahern and others (e.g. Ceci & Bruck, 1995) have voiced about the use of sexualized behavior and describe how the methodology underlying this best practice evaluation model effectively mitigates such concerns. Our goal in this discussion is to affirm the continued use of sexualized behavior as a possible abuse indicator in forensic CSA assessments.

THE LINK BETWEEN SEXUAL ABUSE AND SEXUALIZED BEHAVIOR

Child sexual abuse typically involves an adult or adolescent engaging in sex with a child. The sex can take many forms from voyeurism to oral-genital contact to anal rape. The specific impact of such experiences on children is far from uniform, with persistent harm related to the severity and nature of the abuse, the level of the child's "trauma burden" or prior history of traumatic events, and the response the child receives when the abuse is disclosed or becomes known (Berliner, 2011). Finkelhor and Browne (1985; Finkelhor, 1994) coined the term "traumatic sexualization" to refer to the distortions in sexual attitudes, feelings, cognitions, and behaviors that frequently result from CSA. Finkelhor and Browne also suggested several psychological mechanisms that may underlie traumatic sexualization. In some cases, the mechanisms are inherently destructive. In others, they involve introducing children to normative adult issues for which the child is developmentally ill-prepared. The proposed traumagenic mechanisms include:

1. The child develops misconceptions, false beliefs, and unhealthy attitudes about sex.
2. The child develops an age-inappropriate interest in and preoccupation with sex.
3. Parts of the child's anatomy are fetishized and given distorted importance and meaning.
4. The child learns to expect all or most relationships to have a sexual component.
5. The child receives attention, privileges, or other rewards for sex and learns to use sex as a means for getting needs met or for manipulating others.

6. The child's identity and self-worth become dependent on his or her sexual value to others.
7. The child seeks mastery over feelings of fear and powerlessness by repetition of the negative sexual events.
8. The child develops an aversion to sex and to expressions of affection due to associations with fear, pain, shame, and powerlessness.

The first seven of the mechanisms would lead to higher levels of sexualized behavior among children who have been sexually abused. The last mechanism—aversion to reminders of sex, intimacy, and affection—would lead to *decreased* levels of sexual behavior (see Olafson, this issue, for further discussion of the pervasive effects of CSA across other psychological and behavioral domains).

Early studies using a variety of sexual behavior surveys generally confirmed the prediction of significantly higher levels of sexual behavior among children with histories of sexual abuse compared to those with no such histories (Cavanagh-Johnson, 1993; Cavanagh-Johnson & Friend, 1995; Dubowitz, Black, Harrington, & Veerschoore, 1993; Friedrich, 1993; Kendall-Tackett, Williams, & Finkelhor, 1993). Since the mid-1990s, the most commonly used instrument for assessing sexual behavior in children has been the Child Sexual Behavior Inventory (CSBI) developed by Friedrich (1997). The CSBI is a psychometrically sound, 38-item questionnaire that is usually completed by the child's primary caretaker. The CSBI is designed for children ages 2 to 12 years and provides clinical cutoff scores and individual item norms for both sexes for three different age groups (2–5 years, 6–9 years, 10–12 years). The CSBI also provides clinical and normative data on two subscales: developmentally related sexual behaviors (DRSB; Friedrich, Grambsch, Damon, Hewitt, Kaverola, Lang, Wolfe, & Broughton, 1992) and sexual abuse sensitive items (SASI; Friedrich, 1995, 1997, 2007).

Although there is consensus in the field that sexualized behavior, by itself, should not be the basis for a conclusion of sexual abuse, studies employing the CSBI have typically reported clinically significant levels of sexualized behavior in 30–40% of abused samples (e.g., Friedrich, 1997, 2007; Friedrich, Olafson, & Faller, 2007). Several studies have also reported statistically significant differences between abused and nonabused samples on numerous individual CSBI items (Friedrich, 1997, 2007). The CSBI items differentiating sexually abused from nonabused children predominantly fall in one of the following domains: sexual preoccupation, boundary problems, deviant patterns of masturbation, sexually intrusive behaviors, and precocious sexual interactions with others (Friedrich, 1997). More severe sexual abuse, the use of threats, and more than one perpetrator are associated with higher levels of sexualized behavior across multiple domains (Friedrich et al., 1992). The child's experience of sexual arousal, fear, and pain during the abuse and the perpetrator's use of grooming are associated with more intrusive types of sexual behavior problems (Hall, Mathews, & Pearce, 1998).

In conclusion, the underlying dynamics of child sexual victimization postulated by Finkelhor and Browne (1985) lead to predictions that age-inappropriate sexualized behavior will be one of the adverse outcomes of sexual abuse. Although 30–40% of sexually abused children display such behavior, an additional unknown subset of child victims are likely to exhibit sexual avoidant symptoms that may not be apparent until a later stage of development (Merrill, Guimond, Thomsen, & Milner, 2003) or without specialized assessment techniques (Brilleslijper-Kater & Baartman, 2000; Brilleslijper-Kater, Friedrich & Corwin, 2004).

THE MULTIPLE ROLES OF SEXUAL BEHAVIOR PROBLEMS

Developmentally inappropriate sexual behavior has long been viewed as a useful marker for CSA (Friedrich, 1997; Friedrich et al., 2001; Kendall-Tackett et al., 1993). As a result, sexual behavior problems can potentially serve several functions in the screening, assessment, and decision-making process. Perhaps the most important feature of such function is as a possible screen for identifying children who may have been sexually abused. Such screening has at least two rationales. First, screening is crucial because, though the majority of sexually victimized children do not initiate abuse disclosures during childhood, a subset of these children will disclose if their sexualized behavior results in their being directly questioned (see reviews by London, Bruck, Ceci, Shuman, 2005; Lyon & Ahern, 2011; Paine & Hanson, 2002). Second, research suggests that approximately one-third of children for whom there are strong suspicions of CSA fail to disclose despite skilled interviewing (Hershkowitz, Orbach, Lamb, Sternberg, & Horowitz, 2006, 2007; Lamb, Hershkowitz, Orbach, & Esplin, 2008). An analysis of the severity of reported sexualized behaviors (including SASI items on the CSBI) may aid in identifying a limited subset of these children for follow-up if resources are insufficient for further assessment of all children in this subgroup.

There are at least two functions of sexualized behaviors related to assessment. First, an analysis of both the onset and type of sexual behavior problems and the response of adults to such behaviors may be useful in assessing the *validity* of the child's report of abuse. For example, a first-time onset of sexualized behavior soon after the alleged abusive event may provide corroborative support for the child's account. Conversely, evidence that fear of punishment for being "caught" behaving sexually may have motivated the child's report of abuse could undermine support for the abuse allegation. Second, an analysis of the onset and pattern of sexual behavior problems sometimes suggests hypotheses about the *origin* of the behavior.

For example, a four-year-old's sexualized dancing while using furniture as a "pole" may suggest one type of sexual exposure. Another four-year-old's repeated offers of oral sex to boys on the playground may suggest another. A four-year-old girl's invitation to a preschool classmate to play "daddy and mommy" by sleeping naked under a blanket may suggest an altogether different source of knowledge.

Finally, sexualized behavior frequently plays a role in structured decision making about abuse allegations. Several sets of guidelines have been proposed to aid professionals in decisions about the likelihood of CSA (e.g., Sgroi, Porter, & Blick, 1982; Corwin, 1988; Herman, 1992). These guidelines generally consist of a list of abuse indicators to be counted or weighed in the decision process. Faller (2007) has identified 16 sets of decision-making guidelines, 10 of which include sexualized behavior as evidence of sexual abuse. Among all child behavioral symptoms of sexual abuse, sexualized behavior has the most extensive data on norms for both sexually abused and non-sexually-abused children, and the overall strongest validity in discriminating between these groups (Friedrich, 1997). As a result, sexualized behavior will also likely be incorporated in the future actuarial prediction models recommended by Faust and colleagues (2009a) and Herman (2009).

COMPREHENSIVE FORENSIC EVALUATIONS: CHIC DEFINED

The comprehensive forensic evaluation model (CFE) is one of the most commonly endorsed approaches for assessing allegations of child sexual abuse, especially in complex cases (e.g., APSAC, 1997; Faller, 2007; Kuehnle, 1996, 1998). In this section we highlight a widely used subtype of CFE as a best practice model of forensic assessment because of its responsiveness to many criticisms of current forensic practice, including concerns about the use of sexualized behavior as a possible abuse indicator. The CHIC evaluation model is named for four characteristics which define the model:[1] comprehensive, hypothesis-testing, idiographic, corroborative.

Comprehensive refers to an emphasis on gathering information from a wide range of sources for case decision making. In addition to interviews with the alleged child victim, these sources include agency records, a medical examination, interviews with all parent figures and major caregivers, collateral interviews (e.g., teachers, child care providers), interviews with the alleged abuser, and behavior ratings (e.g., the CSBI) completed by adults who know the child. Psychological testing of the alleged child victim or the alleged abuser is sometimes helpful. The CFE model is enhanced when the evaluation is conducted by a multidisciplinary team (Faller, 2007) or as part of a joint investigation that includes child protective services (CPS) and law enforcement personnel (APSAC, 2002).

Hypothesis-testing refers to identifying and testing multiple plausible explanations for the allegations in the case, ideally with the goal of determining the single explanation that best accounts for the available evidence. Hypothesis-testing drives the assessment process by providing purpose and direction. The most effective hypotheses are case-specific. For example, the primary hypotheses in the evaluation of Cindi, a 10-year-old girl who reportedly disclosed sexual abuse to a classmate are as follows:

1. Cindi was sexually abused by Charles, her mother's boyfriend, as alleged.
2. Cindi was not sexually abused by Charles as alleged, but the classmate intentionally misrepresented Cindi's statements to her.
3. Cindi was not sexually abused by Charles as alleged, but the classmate misunderstood Cindi's statements to her.
4. Cindi was not sexually abused by Charles but is intentionally making a false allegation for secondary gain (e.g., to break up her mother's relationship with Charles).
5. Cindi was sexually abused by someone other than Charles.

Idiographic assessment complements hypothesis-testing methodology and rests on the premise that each case is unique and can be understood only through an analysis of its idiosyncratic elements. An idiographic explanation of the key elements typically takes the form of a highly individualized, descriptive narrative (Thornton, 2008, 2010). Constructing such a case-specific narrative requires gathering, organizing, and analyzing information from a variety of sources unique to the case. The completed case narrative is compared against the hypotheses. The hypothesis that most closely matches the case narrative is viewed as most likely valid.

Corroborative refers to an emphasis on obtaining independent verification of substantive evidence in the case. Sources for such verification may include agency records, independent witnesses, or the perspectives of non-involved individuals. The degree of corroboration is a factor in determining the weight given to substantive evidence.

Although the CHIC evaluation model is likely the most popular comprehensive model in use today, other variations exist, defined by the combination of hypothesis-testing, idiographic, and corroborative characteristics employed. One such assessment approach whose relevance to our appraisal of sexualized behavior will later become apparent relies on nomothetic rather than idiographic methodology. Nomothetic methodology downplays the uniqueness of individual cases and emphasizes commonality among cases (Gelles, 1982; Ponterotto, 2005). Case decisions are made on the basis of comparisons to broadly applied, external criteria such as structured decision guidelines, symptom norms, or actuarial methods. In the case of 10-year-old Cindi, a forensic evaluator using a nomothetic approach would focus on whether Cindi meets several criteria common to sexually abused children, not on whether her case narrative is coherent in explaining the known case facts.

Consistent with a nomothetic approach, several sets of guidelines for deciding the likelihood of sexual abuse have been proposed (e.g., Corwin, 1988; Faller, 2003, 2007; Gardner, 1987, 1992; Jones & McGraw, 1987; Sgroi, Porter, and Blick, 1982). Although not referencing idiographic and nomothetic terminology, Kuehnle (1998) has proposed a hybrid evaluation model that attempts to combine the best features of both.

To a considerable degree, the CHIC evaluation model evolved in response to criticism of other evaluative approaches (Faller, 2007). Consequently, as we shall see, CHIC methodology offers ready remedies for several of the concerns expressed by Poole and Wolfe (2009) and Faust et al. (2009a, 2009b).

CONCERNS ABOUT THE DIAGNOSTIC VALUE OF SEXUAL BEHAVIOR PROBLEMS

The general argument against the use of sexual behavior problems in the forensic process, articulated in part by Faust et al. (2009a, 2009b) and Poole and Wolfe (2009), can be succinctly summarized: The diagnostic value of sexualized behavior in CSA assessments is overrated. Forensic evaluators who rely on sexualized behavior are likely to overestimate the strength of the evidence in support of abuse. This will lead to a large number of false allegations of sexual abuse being mistakenly substantiated as true.

This argument is built on a number of premises, including several with which we take issue. In this section, we outline these premises and critique their validity and relevance in light of current forensic practice:

1. **There is substantial research evidence that sexual curiosity and sexual behavior is normal, even among very young children (cf. Poole & Wolfe, 2009)**.

    Our response:

    Some forms of sexual curiosity and sexual behavior are common in childhood; others are atypical and even aberrant. The research summarized by Poole and Wolfe (2009) suggests that self-stimulation and reciprocal looking at and touching genitals, for example, are common among preschool-age children. The research is less clear about the frequency of "simulated intercourse" prior to age 12 (Davies, Glaser, & Kossoff, 2000; Friedrich, Grambsch, Broughton, Kuiper, & Beilke, 1991, Friedrich, Fisher, Broughton, Houston, & Shafran, 1998). However, more intrusive sexual behavior involving aggression, vaginal or anal penetration, and oral-genital contact are rarely reported prior to age 12 (Friedrich et al., 1991, 1998). The CSBI makes a critical distinction between normative sexual behaviors that are grouped in the Developmentally Related Sexual Behaviors (DRSB) subscale and sexual behaviors that may be associated with sexual abuse and are categorized in the Sexual Abuse Specific Items (SASI) subscale. Several of the SASI behaviors are associated with likelihood ratios of 20:1 or greater, suggesting "strong" evidence of abuse. In Friedrich's (2001) research, for example, the prevalence of "pretending dolls have sex" during everyday play activities was 23% among preschool age girls with histories of CSA but only 1% among nonabused preschoolers, producing a 23:1 likelihood odds ratio.

Equally important, the comprehensive assessment and the hypothesis testing methodology of CHIC evaluations provides an opportunity for assessing a number of alternative explanations for the child's sexual behavior, including the possibility that the behavior in question falls within normal limits or is derived from an experience other than sexual abuse.

2. **Caregiver reports of child behavior problem including sexual behaviors are known to be unreliable, inaccurate, and often biased (cf. Poole & Wolfe, 2009).**
   Our response:
   Poole and Wolfe rightly point out that the CSBI and many other methods of data gathering that rely on caretaker report may not be accurate. Caretakers view and report their children's behavior through their own lenses, which reflect their life experiences and their beliefs about the probability of sexual abuse (Poole & Wolfe, 2009). Honest memory errors also occur, while deliberate reporting errors to manipulate or mislead are infrequently made (Trocmé & Bala, 2005). Forensic evaluators can minimize the impact of such reporting errors and biases by seeking corroboration from independent sources including teachers, other professionals, and disinterested collaterals. The CHIC evaluation model includes an explicit expectation that substantive evidence used in case decisions should be corroborated. Evidence lacking independent verification is weighed accordingly.

3. **There are no diagnostic behavior indicators of sexual abuse, including aberrant sexualized behavior, that occur in all or even most abused children while being simultaneously absent in all nonabused children (Ceci & Bruck, 1995; cf. Poole & Wolfe, 2009).**
   Our response:
   This is not a realistic standard for judging the validity or utility of a diagnostic indicator (Faust et al., 2009a). Diagnostic criteria across a range of medical or psychological conditions could not meet such a standard. Faust and associates (2009a) use the example of dissociative identity disorder (DID) to make the point that a variable may be a valid indication of CSA even if it applies to only a small minority of sexual abuse victims. If a small

percentage of abuse victims develop the disorder who would otherwise not have developed it, then there is a valid and possibly discriminating relationship between DID and sexual abuse, despite the rarity of DID on the whole (Faust et al., 2009a). A symptom such as dissociative identity disorder is not used in isolation but is weighted with other signs and symptoms in the CSA assessment process. Similarly, sexual behavior problems are combined with other indicators to make a determination about the validity of a CSA allegation. The CHIC model encourages a comprehensive search for evidence relevant to the allegation to minimize decision-making dependency on any single abuse indicator.

4. **Research has shown that sexualized behavior in children may result from a number of sources other than sexual abuse (cf. Poole & Wolfe, 2009).**

Our response:

We concur with Poole & Wolfe (2009) that this research finding warrants repeated emphasis. Sexual abuse is only one of several possible origins of age-inappropriate sexual behavior in children. Friedrich (1997; Friedrich et al., 1998; Friedrich, Trane, & Gully, 2005) collected normative data on the sexual behavior of more than 2,000 children. Although sexual abuse was the factor most frequently associated with elevated levels of sexualized behavior, the second most common associated factor was family sexuality including exposure to adult nudity, sexual materials, and sexual activities. Friedrich and others have identified a third subgroup of children exhibiting precocious or aberrant sexual knowledge and behavior who have no known histories of sexual abuse or sexual exposure (Drach, Wientzen, & Ricci, 2001; Friedrich, 1997; Friedrich et al., 2001; Tarren-Sweeney, 2008). Common factors among these children include family stress, domestic violence, physical abuse, and psychiatric disturbances. Sexualized behavior among this third subset of children may represent self-soothing behaviors, problems in emotional and behavioral self-regulation, or undetected sexual abuse or sexual exposure as noted earlier. The consensus in the field of forensic CSA assessment is that the presence of developmentally inappropriate sexual behaviors is insufficient to support a conclusion of CSA (e.g., Association for the Treatment of Sexual Abusers, 2006; Chaffin, Letourneau, & Silvosky, 2002), an opinion held by Friedrich (e.g. Friedrich, 1997; Friedrich et al., 2005). The methodology of the CHIC evaluation model is well-suited to develop and test alternative hypotheses related to the origin of sexualized behavior.

5. **Reported differences in the rates of sexualized behavior in abused and nonabused children are likely exaggerated because of sampling biases (cf. Poole & Wolfe, 2009).**

Our response:

One such potential sampling bias that Poole & Wolfe (2009) identify is the probability that children who act out sexually are more likely to be questioned by parents and professional about possible CSA. If sexualized behavior increases the likelihood that sexual abuse will be discovered, children who have been abused may be overrepresented among those children whose sexualized behavior is discovered, even if abused and nonabused children do not actually differ overall in sexualized behavior (Lyon & Koehler, 1996). A second source of bias is the possibility that once CSA is discovered, parents and professionals may watch the child more carefully for sexualized behavior and may therefore misinterpret normal sexual play as aberrant or precocious (Lyon & Koehler, 1996). A third source of bias may be the use of circular reasoning by some researchers who may categorize children as sexually abused on the basis of sexualized behavior and then conclude that sexually abused children exhibit more sexualized behavior (Drach et al., 2001).

These three sources of possible distortion in the differential rates of sexual behavior problems among abused and nonabused children represent a significant challenge to forensic evaluators relying on nomothetic assessment procedures. However, CHIC evaluations using idiographic methodology do not depend on precise estimates of differential symptom rates between abused and nonabused children for their case decisions but rather integrate sexual behavior findings with other information and use it as corroborative.

6. When population base rates are taken into account, the diagnostic value of sexualized behavior as an abuse indicator is minimal (Faust et al., 2009a).

Our response:

The base rate argument has long been used to challenge the validity of forensic decision making (e.g., Poole & Lamb, 1998; Wood, 1996). Our intention here is to explain the argument fairly, then refute it decisively. The argument is highly mathematical, so explaining then dismissing it is a lengthy process. Plus, we will attempt to do so first using a traditional Bayesian approach and then using a simplified approach for the mathematically avoidant reader.

The base rate argument derives from application of Bayes' Theorem to forensic decision making (Poole & Lamb, 1998; Proeve, 2008; Wood, 1996). According to Bayes' Theorem, the diagnostic accuracy of decisions based on an abuse indicator like sexualized behavior involves a combination of two sets of probabilities or odds: (a) the likelihood that a sexually abused child will exhibit the behavior compared with the likelihood that a nonabused child will exhibit it (aka the likelihood ratio) and (b) the base rate of sexually abused children in the target population versus the base rate of nonabused children (Faust et al., 2009a).

An example will illustrate the logic of Bayes' Theorem: Suppose the base rate of sexual abuse in the target population (e.g., all school-aged children in county X) is 10%. The base rate odds, or the likelihood of any given school-aged child having been sexually abused, are therefore 10:90 or 1:9. Base rate odds of 1:9 mean that one of every 10 children (1 + 9) has been sexually abused and that there are nine nonabused children for every one abused child. Suppose the relevant abuse indicator is a sexual behavior that is exhibited by 16% of school-aged sexually abused children but in only 2% of nonabused children. This translates into a "likelihood ratio" of 16:2 or 8:1. In other words, exhibiting this behavior increases the odds of abuse by eight times. The presence of this sexualized behavior may initially seem like substantial evidence of CSA. However, to accurately assess the diagnostic value of the sexual behavior in this population, we must multiply the base rate odds by the likelihood ratio: As we can see, 1:9 (base rate odds) x 8:1 (likelihood ratio) gives us 8:9 odds of abuse. Therefore, eight out of every 17 children (8 + 9) who exhibit the sexualized behavior, or only 47%, have actually been abused. Thus, a child in this target population who exhibits the sexualized behavior has only a 47% probability of having been sexually abused. This represents poor diagnostic accuracy for the sexualized behavior in this case. One could repeat these Bayesian calculations with a number of different sexualized behaviors and obtain similar, low-level probabilities of abuse. Faust and his associates argue that because of the substantial disparity in base rates between abused and nonabused children in nearly all realistic populations, a single abuse indicator such as a sexualized behavior has little diagnostic value (Bridges et al., 2009; Faust et al., 2009a). In this example, the base rate disparity is 1:9. In other populations, the disparity may be as high as 1:19. Such base rates swamp the diagnostic power of most single abuse indicators, leaving the indicator impotent. Faust and colleauges (2009a) therefore claim overwhelming validation for their first proposition that when population base rates are taken into account, the diagnostic value of most abuse indicators is minimal.

We concede this point but contend the point is inconsequential. A 47% probability of abuse based on a single sexualized behavior is neither surprising nor disconcerting. As noted earlier, it is the consensus of the field that sexualized behavior is not conclusive evidence of sexual abuse (Chaffin et al., 2002; Friedrich, 2002; Friedrich et al., 2005). Such behavior must be considered or combined with other evidence for a case decision. We would therefore not expect a single indicator, on its own, to reliably differentiate abused from nonabused children. In other words, responsible professionals do not conduct forensic assessment in the way that Faust and his associates imply that they do. The irrelevance of their base rate argument to actual practice is clearer when we add a second point.

The second part of our response is to assert that the use of multiple indicators trumps the impact of base rates (Proeve, 2009). Specifically, we offer a hypothetical case example to demonstrate the diagnostic power of a small number of independent (noncorrelated) abuse indicators in overcoming significant base rate disparities.

Case Example

An anonymous report is made to CPS that John Smith, a registered sex offender whose parole conditions mandate no contact with children, is living in the home of Sarah and her mother. A criminal record check confirms Mr. Smith's sex offender and parole status, and a joint CPS/law enforcement investigation is launched. Sarah, age 7, is interviewed, but reveals nothing of concern. Sarah's mother denies any possibility of inappropriate actions on John's part because Sarah has never been left alone with him. Mr. Smith confirms the mother's denials of accessibility. Sarah's mother also reports strict rules regarding nudity in the home, no access to sexually explicit materials, and no possibility of Sarah being exposed to adult sexual activities. However, the investigation reveals one concerning behavior by Sarah. Her teacher reports that on two occasions during the month since Christmas vacation, Sarah has exposed her genitals to other girls in the restroom—a behavior very uncharacteristic of Sarah.

Given this evidence alone, how concerned should the CPS investigator be about possible sexual abuse? How much should the level of concern increase if more evidence is added? We will first discuss Sarah's case using a traditional Bayesian approach. Next, we will present a simplified Bayesian approach for readers who are less mathematically inclined.

Traditional Bayesian Approach

According to Friedrich's (1997) norms for girls in Sarah's age range, 14% of sexually abused girls exhibit this behavior, but only 2% of nonabused girls do so. This likelihood ratio is 14 ÷ 2 or 7:1. This ratio means that Sarah's sexualized behavior increases the likelihood of abuse by 7 times, indicating moderate diagnostic power. As we have noted, however, the likelihood ratio by itself provides a misleading estimate of the strength of the evidence. The base rate of abuse from the appropriate population must first be factored in.

At least two populations are potentially relevant. Identifying the correct population is essential because the base rate of abuse is likely substantially lower in general populations than in populations referred for CSA assessment. If we were estimating the diagnostic value of abuse indicators used at the screening level, the relevant population would be the general population of children in which the screening occurred. In Sarah's case, this general population would likely be defined as either all the children in Sarah's school, her county, or her state. Because our case scenario involves assessing the diagnostic value of indicators in the evaluation phase, the relevant population includes only children referred for assessment of CSA. As a result, children involved in CPS investigations of CSA in Sarah's county agency would likely comprise the appropriate population.

Accurate estimates of base rates are seldom available. However, in this case, the substantiation rate of sexual abuse cases in the CPS agency conducting Sarah's investigation might be a realistic proxy. We will use 17% as a conservative estimate of the substantiation rate/base rate of CSA to be consistent with the Bayesian example used by Faust and colleagues (2009a). This means that the probability is only about 1 out of 5 (.17/.83 = .20) that a child randomly selected from the CPS caseloads of this fictional agency is truly abused. According to Bayes' Theorem, the base rate represents the prior probability of abuse, before any evidence is applied. The probability of abuse after evidence is added is estimated by multiplying the base rate odds by the likelihood ratio of the evidence. Thus, 1:5 multiplied by 7:1 equals 7:5. The product, in this case, 7:5 is then turned into a probability: 58% or 7 of every 12 children in this CPS sample who expose their genitals to other children would likely have been abused. Thus, when the population base rates are factored in, it is clear that the probability of abuse based on the limited evidence available is quite low.

However, regardless of whether the CPS investigator adjusted for the base rates, substantiating sexual abuse on the basis of sexualized behavior alone would not be considered accepted practice. More evidence would be needed. Nonabuse origins of the sexualized behavior would have to be considered. As a result, fears of a false substantiation in a case such as this because the evaluator did not consider population base rates are unfounded, and error estimates based on such fears are likely exaggerated.

Let's suppose that the CPS and law inforcement investigators in this case expanded their efforts and conducted a more comprehensive investigation. The investigators also expand the set of hypotheses to be examined, including adding the possible hypothesis that Sarah was sexually abused but is fearful or reluctant to disclose because of Mr. Smith's continued access to her. His access is subsequently restricted. Sarah and her mother are both reinterviewed and additional collaterals are contacted.

During her second interview, Sarah provides a detailed description of several episodes of sexual abuse by John that began during Christmas vacation when her mom was out shopping. The abuse took the form of John fondling Sarah's genitals and forcing her to masturbate him. Sarah did not inform her mother of the abuse because of threats by John. Sarah admits that she frequently thinks about what happened, partly because of guilt that some of what John did felt pleasurable. She recounts that the two times she got in trouble at school for "trying to talk to other girls" about private parts occurred when she could not get thoughts of her abuse out of her mind. In her second interview, Sarah's mother admits that Sarah's behavior has changed substantially since John moved in just before the holidays. Sarah has become moody and depressed and spends most of the time now locked in her room. The mother attributes these changes to Sarah being jealous of the time she and John spend together. Sarah's after-school teacher reports that Sarah has been a markedly different child since returning from the Christmas break four weeks ago. From a gregarious, highly motivated student, Sarah has become introspective, often daydreaming for 15–20 minutes at a time, especially as the time to go home draws near. Sarah's maternal grandmother also comments about Sarah's recent "funk." When asked about child care arrangements, she describes two occasions during the holidays when she stopped by unannounced and found John alone with Sarah.

Table 1 shows the math and effect of adding additional behavior indicators on the probability of abuse. The probability of abuse prior to adding any evidence is 17%, or the base rate of sexual abuse in the CPS sample. Introduction of the first abuse indication increases the probability of abuse to 58% (step 1). The next indicator that we add is Sarah's disclosure. To estimate the likelihood ratio of her disclosure, let's assume a disclosure rate of 40% among children sexually abused but who have not made a prior disclosure (Lyon, 2007). We assume a 5% false disclosure rate, which is likely high but has some support (Everson & Boat, 1989). Thus a conservative estimate of the likelihood ratio for a disclosure of sexual abuse by a sexually abused child in such a case is 40 ÷ 5, or 8 to 1. This means that Sarah's disclosure increases the odds of abuse by 8 times. According to Bayes' Theorem, an iterative process is followed to estimate the augmenting value of each piece of new evidence. The existing posterior odds (e.g., step 1) are multiplied by the likelihood odds of each piece of new evidence. The resulting product gives the new posterior odds, based on the addition of the new evidence. Thus, with the addition of Sarah's disclosure to the sexual behavior indicator, "shows sex parts," the probability of abuse has jumped to 92%.

Sarah's case at first appears to be a target-rich environment for behavior indicators of possible CSA. However, many of the remaining indicators are

TABLE 1 Traditional Bayesian Theorem Demonstration of Impact of Multiple Indicators

	Hypothetical CPS sample		
	Abused	Nonabused	Probabilty of abuse
Base rate odds of CSA (.17 to .83)	1	5	1/6 = 17%
Likelihood ratio of abuse, given "shows sex parts to children" (.14 to.02)	x 7	x 1	
Odds of abuse, given "shows sex parts"	7	5	7/12 = 58% (step 1)
Likelihood ratio of abuse, given disclosure (.40 to .05)	x 8	x 1	
Odds of abuse, given "shows sex parts" + disclosure	56	5	56/61 = 92% (step 2)
Likelihood ratio of abuse, given "significant behavior change" (.66 to .07)	x 9	x 1	
Odds of abuse, given "shows sex parts" + disclosure + "significant behavior changes"	504	5	504/509 = 99% (step 3)

likely redundant or significantly correlated and thus may be limited in their contribution to the decision process. For example, "moody," "depressed," "spends a lot of time in her room," and in a "funk" are likely related to the same behavior domain. "Introspective," "spacing out," and "daydreaming" are also likely correlated behaviors and so cannot be entered into the Bayesian formula as separate independent indicators. Both sets of behaviors, however, can be categorized as a significant change in behavior reported by the mother, grandmother, and after-school teacher. A study comparing sexually abused and nonabused girls Sarah's age found a 66% to 7% prevalence rate of demonstrated a "significant behavior change" (Wells, McCann, Adams, Voris, & Ensign, 1995). This prevalence is associated with a moderate likelihood ratio of 9:1. As is shown in Table 1, when this second behavior indicator is added at Step 3, the probability of Sarah having been sexually abused jumps to 99%. In other words, in this CPS sample, 99 out of 100 children who expose their genital to other children and make a first time disclosure of sexual abuse and exhibit a significant behavior or personality change would likely be abused.

Faust and colleagues (2009a) dismiss the import and impact of multiple indicators, stating that a "ceiling" on predictive accuracy is usually reached after the addition of three to five nonredundant indicators. Sarah's case illustrates their point exactly. We reach a "ceiling" of 99% probability with the addition of only three, presumably nonredundant indicators.

However, one might object that sexualized behavior and disclosure may not be independent as previously advertised. Perhaps nonabused children when questioned are more likely to make false claims of abuse in order to justify or excuse their sexual behavior. In such a case, the 99% final probability would have to be adjusted downward. Note, however, that we have yet to consider John's status as a registered sex offender as a risk factor for Sarah (conservatively, a likelihood ratio of at least 2:1). Nor have we factored in substantial idiosyncratic evidence that corroborates Sarah's disclosure statement. This evidence includes:

A. Corroboration by the grandmother of Sarah's claim of having been left alone with the alleged perpetrator despite his and her mother's denial
B. Corroboration by her after-school teacher of Sarah's report of intrusive thinking
C. Corroboration of Sarah's report of the initial occurrence of the abuse (during the Christmas vacation) by the report of behavior changes noted by her mother, grandmother, and teachers
D. A logical connection between Sarah's description of the abuse and her sexualized behavior at school

By restricting the definition of "disclosure" to include only certain types of disclosures, we can factor in the independent corroboration of two essential elements of Sarah's disclosure (being left alone with the alleged abuser and the initiation of the abuse during Christmas vacation). The new disclosure variable would be defined as "disclosure with independent corroboration of at least two key elements." Introducing the new definition would likely have two effects: (a) to increase the likelihood ratio for the disclosure variable from 8:1 to 16:1 or better and (b) to reduce, if not eliminate, the possible nonindependence of the sexualized behavior and disclosure variables.

In Sarah's case, it is therefore safe to conclude that three to five abuse indictors result in a 99 % + probability of abuse—and we still have unused abuse indicators. This case illustrates the contribution of a detailed disclosure elicited by a well-trained interviewer. Such a disclosure often produces a mother lode of disclosure elements that substantially increase the likelihood ratio for disclosure. "Disclosure of abuse" could be redefined as "disclosure with elements A, B, C and X, Y, Z." If this definition were expanded to include independent corroboration of several of the essential elements, one could virtually eliminate false positive "disclosures" among nonabused children, thereby increasing the likelihood ratio of the disclosure variable exponentially.

Simplified Bayesian Approach

Part of the difficulty of understanding the traditional Bayesian approach is the use of terms such as *odds, likelihood ratios*, and *posterior probabilities* that are unfamiliar to many readers. These terms can be avoided if we track the impact of additional indicators using children rather than odds. Table 2 presents Sarah's case as the percentage of abused and nonabused children exhibiting Sarah's pattern of behavior at each stage of the Bayesian model. The agreed on base rate of 17% of abused children means that 170 out of 1,000 children in a hypothetical CPS sample in Sarah's county would be abused and 830 would be nonabused. The frequency of "shows sex parts to children" is 14% among abused children and 2% among nonabused children. Therefore, only 23.8 of the 170 abused children we started with at the base rate can be expected to exhibit this behavior (14% of 170 children), while 16.6 of the 830 nonabused children we started with can be expected to exhibit the behavior (2% of 830 children). Applying the same logic, 9.5 of the abused children who exhibited "shows sex parts" can be expected to make a disclosure of abuse (40% of 23.5), while only .83 of a child in the nonabused group can be expected to exhibit the sexual behavior, plus disclose (5% of 16.6). Similarly, when the third abuse indicator, "significant behavior change," with a frequency of 66% among abused children and 7% in nonabused children is introduced at step 3, 6.28 abused children and only .06 of a nonabused child can be expected to exhibit all three indicators (66% of 9.5 versus 7% of .83) This means that in the hypothetical CPS sample of 1,000 children, there will be 6.28 truly abused children who exhibit all three

TABLE 2 Simplified Bayesian Theorem Demonstration of Impact of Multiple Indicators

Hypothetical CPS sample of 1000 accepted referrals			
	Abused	Nonabused	Probabilty of abuse
Base rate of CSA (17%)	170	830	170/1000 = 17% (base rate)
Frequency of "show sex parts to children" (14% vs. 2%)	x .14	x .02	
Number of children who "show sex parts"	23.8	16.6	23.8/40.4 = 58% (step 1)
Frequency of disclosure (40% vs. 5%)	x .40	x .05	
Number of children who "show sex parts" + disclosure	9.5	.83	9.5/10.3 = 92% (step 2)
Frequency of "significant Behavior change" (66% vs. 7%)	x .66	x .07	
Number of children who "show sex parts" + disclosure + "significant behavior changes"	6.28	.06	6.28/6.34 = 99% (step 3)
Number of children who "show sex parts: + disclosure	x16.67	x 16.67	
+ "significant behavior changes" after recalibration of nonabused group to 1.0	104.7	1.0	104.7/105.7 = 99% (recalibration)

abuse indicators that Sarah exhibits and only .06 of a nonabused child who exhibits all three behaviors. Since .06 of a child is an impossible statistic, it is useful to recalibrate the .06 of a child to 1 child. This can be done by multiplying the 6.28 abused children and the .06 nonabused children by 16.67. Thus, for every 104 abused children who demonstrate all three indicators (6.28 x 16.67), there is only 1 nonabused child who does so (.06 x 16.67). As shown in Table 2, exhibiting all three indicators as Sarah does means a probability of sexual abuse of over 99%.

We suggest two take-home messages from this discussion. First, the use of multiple indicators clearly trumps the impact of base rates. Three to five *nonredundant* abuse indicators of only moderate strength are sufficient to overcome the differential base rates of abused and nonabused children in most realistic samples. The fact that the introduction of additional indicators is an iterative, multiplicative process accounts for the powerful impact of multiple indicators on abuse probabilities. The second take-home message is that despite its use by Faust and colleagues (Bridges et al., 2009, Faust et al., 2009a) to criticize, Bayes' Theorem is actually quite supportive of forensic practice (see also Lyon, Ahern, & Scurich, this issue, for further discussion of the misuse of Bayes' Theorem to discredit forensic practice). More important, Bayes' Theorem provides us with the math and the logic to demonstrate the extreme probative value of three or more abuse indicators of even only moderate diagnostic value—as long as the abuse indicators are reasonably independent or noncorrelated. Despite Bayes' Theorem's support for the strategy and logic underlying comprehensive forensic assessment, we must offer a word of caution about its application to specific substantiation decisions. In reality, we do not have sufficiently valid and generalizable estimates of base rates or likelihood ratios to apply a Bayesian approach to actual case decision making. The math and logic are sound; the application is weak.

One final note: Application of Bayesian Theorem to forensic CSA assessments is exclusively a nomothetic process. At each step, group frequencies are used to assess the strength of the abuse indicator being introduced. In addition, the process ends with a single probability, an end point completely void of any of the case's idiosyncratic features.

7. **Abuse indicators like sexualized behavior that have been used in the screening process have limited remaining diagnostic value and should not be reused in the evaluation phase (Bridges et al., 2009).**
   Our response:

Double-dipping is defined as "the unwarranted duplicative use of variables in sexual abuse evaluations" (Bridges et al., 2009, p. 28). It occurs when an abuse indicator is used first during screening for possible abuse, then again during the diagnostic or evaluative phase. Bridges and colleagues (2009) condemn double-dipping as a "surprisingly insidious and destructive practice" that they view as likely "widespread" among forensic evaluators (p. 28).

According to Bridges and colleagues (2009), the problem lies in the fact that, unbeknownst to the evaluator, the indicator uses up its value for *differentiating* abused from nonabused children in the screening phase and has no discriminating value left for the evaluation phase. As an example, Bridges and colleagues (2009) use a hypothetical case in which sexualized behavior is the primary reason children are referred to a clinic for evaluation. In such a case, sexualized behavior has no remaining diagnostic value for discriminating between abused and nonabused children in the evaluation sample because, by selection, every child in the sample acts out sexually. The evaluator who is unaware of this common characteristic of all children in his or her caseload may mistakenly conclude that they were all sexually abused based on sexual acting out without seeking or considering more valid criteria.

The double-dipping argument potentially has serious implications for our field. If an abuse indicator exhibited by a child is used at all in the screening decision to refer the child for evaluation or investigation, then, as the argument goes, the indicator has reduced diagnostic value for that child and should not be used in the child's evaluation. Should this argument be allowed to stand, it could be used to undermine much of the probative evidence in child sexual abuse cases. Fortunately, Lyon and colleagues (this issue) aptly address the issue of double-dipping as it relates to the child's disclosure of abuse. We will address the double-dipping argument as it relates to a broad range of possible abuse indicators.

Let's begin with a case example to demonstrate the gravity of the threat: During her medical workup for "stomach aches," it is discovered that 12-year-old Maria is 12 weeks pregnant. On the basis of her age and pregnancy status, Maria is referred for a forensic assessment. In her interview Maria adamantly denies any sexual contact as well as any knowledge of how she became pregnant. There is therefore no disclosure, and there appear to be no other signs, symptoms, or indicators of abuse other than the pregnancy. DNA testing has revealed no matches among the several males in Maria's life. One might argue that pregnancy in a girl so young is definitive evidence of sexual abuse and no evaluation is needed. Thus far, however, given the facts of the case, we cannot rule out the hypothesis of "consensual" sexual intercourse with a boy her age. Based on the double-dipping argument, it would seem that the evaluator would not be able to use the pregnancy in the diagnostic process because the pregnancy was used in screening and has therefore lost its diagnostic value. Minus the pregnancy, there is no evidence of sexual abuse or even sexual contact. Therefore, the evaluator can look forward to explaining to Maria and her parents that, statistically speaking, Maria's pregnancy doesn't count, so unless they have other symptoms to report, the case will be closed.

Such an outcome is outrageous. But what is the flaw in the double-dipping argument? We submit that there are at least two. Both undermine the relevance of the double-dipping problem to forensic assessment. First, the use of a CHIC evaluation model allows the problem of "the duplicative use of variables" in the screening and evaluation phases to be sidestepped. This sidestepping involves a paradigm shift that occurs between the two phases that transforms the role of abuse indicators in the screening versus the evaluation phase.

The screening process is designed to address the question "Does this child make the cut?" Answering this question for each child involves comparing the child's presenting symptoms to a set of general principles, norms, or criteria that aid in discriminating between likely abused and likely nonabused children. Such a process is nomothetic in nature. In Maria's case, the operative general guideline would likely be "Pregnancy among preadolescents is a high risk factor for sexual abuse." Maria meets this criterion and therefore warrants a referral for further evaluation.

In contrast to screening, the CHIC evaluation is primarily idiographic in nature. The paradigm shift from the nomothetic screening phase to idiographic evaluation phase represents a fundamental transformation in the role of abuse indicators. As a result, double-dipping is no longer an issue. The indicators in the CHIC evaluation are used less to compare and contrast children than to shed light on one child's story. Maria's pregnancy is no longer used to distinguish Maria from the other children in the screening cohort so that she makes the "cut." Instead, the pregnancy is an event (and, in this case, the primary event) to be explained in the narrative. Whether preadolescent pregnancy has a likelihood ratio for predicting CSA of 50 to 1 or 5 to 1 is of minimal relevancy. The abuse indicator's value in the idiographic evaluation phase is only partly dependent on its diagnostic value in discriminating between abused and nonabused children but primarily on its role in, or contribution to, the narrative that is developed.

In Maria's case, the narrative might take many forms. For example, in spreading a broad net to capture relevant information, suppose the evaluator learns that Maria's 60-year-old uncle had visited three months prior to the discovery of her pregnancy, that he left abruptly, and uncharacteristically he has had no contact with the family since. The mother also reports that Maria was emotionally distraught and withdrawn for a few days around the time of his sudden departure. The mother also found blood in Maria's panties at that time, which she interpreted as spotting from Maria's first menstrual period. Maria's family, friends, and teachers rule out the likelihood of a boyfriend. A psychological assessment reveals PTSD symptoms, but no reported traumatic event. As is readily apparent, a narrative emerges from the evaluation data that provides guidance for a follow-up interview with Maria as well as a rationale for interviews with Maria's four female cousins who have had extensive contact with the uncle.

CHIC methodology includes a second feature that undermines the relevance of the double-dipping argument. The diagnostic values of the indicators used at screening are often enhanced during the forensic evaluation phase by a process akin to separating wheat from chaff. Consider that abuse indicators like sexual behavior problems come in at least three levels of specificity: *survey-level* indicators, *screening-level* indicators, and *evaluation-level* indicators. The CSBI (Friedrich, 1997) and the Child Behavior Checklist (Achenbach, 1991) are examples of two paper-and-pencil surveys that yield survey-level data on behavior indicators. Such surveys provide a methodology for efficiently collecting normative data from large samples on an extensive array of behaviors. As a result, the prevalences and likelihood ratios used in Bayesian Theorem illustrations are often taken from their norms. However, the survey items are subject to substantial idiosyncratic interpretation by survey-takers. For example, the CSBI item "masturbates with hand" yields prevalences of 22.6 for sexually abused girls and 5.3 nonabused girls in the 6–9 age range. That said, the term "masturbate" is open to substantial interpretation, from a quick touch to extensive rubbing with sweating and sound effects. In addition, frequency reports of "once in the prior six months" and "several times daily" are counted as equivalent. As a result, estimates of the ability of survey-level indicators to discriminate between abused and nonabused children are likely very inaccurate. In contrast, screening level indicators are likely to be more directly assessed, at least by phone interview so that the terminology would be more consistent across reporters. Thresholds to be counted as a "case" would also likely be higher. "A report of excessive masturbation" might be sufficient to make the cut, but a single brief occurrence of genital rubbing almost six months ago would be promptly screened out. As the imprecise survey-level variables become more focused at the screening level, the diagnostic utility of the indicators is likely to increase.

Evaluation-level indicators would require still higher standards to be considered valid, reliable, and relevant for the evaluation phase. The forensic evaluator would seek an explicit behavioral description of a reported indicator like "excessive masturbation" as well as information on the frequency, severity, timing, and location of occurrence of the behavior. The evaluator would assess the likely reliability of the reporter and any evidence or motivation for bias. If the indicator were considered to have potential significant probative value in the case, the forensic evaluator would likely seek independent corroboration. As part of assessing how the indicator fits within the case narrative, the evaluator would consider the likely cause or meaning of the abuse indicator. For example, so-called excessive masturbation by a four-year-old girl might represent (a) an anxious parent's misinterpretation of normative levels of genital self-stimulation by the child, (b) the child scratching a chronic genital rash that is benign, (c) the child scratching a chronic genital rash caused by a sexually transmitted disease, or (d) orgasmic masturbation by a child re-creating the pleasurable sensations experienced during her earlier sexual abuse. As an outcome of this culling and refining process, the discriminating value of surviving indicators is often substantially enhanced. The indicators in effect become highly reliable and specific. There is therefore no diminution of diagnostic validity from screening to evaluative phases because the indicators themselves have been transformed along the way.

In summary, the double-dipping problem described by Faust and associates does not pose a significant obstacle to the use of sexualized behavior and other abuse indicators in CHIC forensic evaluations.

CONCLUSIONS

We believe this discussion supports the continued use of sexualized behavior as a possible CSA indicator, especially in forensic evaluations employing the CHIC comprehensive model. The methodology underlying CHIC evaluations is well designed to address common threats to the diagnostic utility of sexualized behavior in CSA assessments. This methodology includes the use of a broad range of information sources for a comprehensive search for evidence supporting or refuting the allegations, weighing substantive evidence based on the degree of corroboration, the testing of alternatives hypotheses, and the construction of a case-specific narrative to account for the available evidence. Such a methodology is also likely to increase the likelihood of a balanced evaluation that emphasizes reducing both false positive and false negative errors (Everson & Sandoval, 2011). Achieving a balanced emphasis in forensic assessments on both sensitivity and specificity is a worthy goal.

NOTE

1. This model is very similar to others described in the literature (e.g., Faller, 2007; Kuehnle, 1996).

REFERENCES

Achenbach, T. (1991). *Manual for the child behavior checklist/4–18 and 1991 profile*. Burlington, VT: University of Vermont Department of Psychiatry.

American Professional Society on the Abuse of Children. (1997). *Guidelines for psychosocial evaluation of suspected sexual abuse in children* (2nd ed.) Elmhurst, IL: Author.

American Professional Society on the Abuse of Children. (2002). *Guidelines on investigative interviewing in cases of alleged child abuse*. Elmhurst, IL: Author.

Association for the Treatment of Sexual Abusers. (2006). Report of task force on sexual behavior problems. *Child Maltreatment, 13*(2), 199–218.

Berliner, L. (2011). Child sexual abuse: Definitions, prevalence and consequences. In J. Myers (Ed.), *APSAC handbook on child maltreatment,* (3rd ed., pp. 215–232). Thousand Oaks: Sage.

Bridges, A., Faust, D., & Ahern, D. (2009). Methods for the identification of sexually abused children. In K. Kuehnle & M. Connell (Eds.), *The evaluation of child sexual abuse allegations: A comprehensive guide to assessment and testimony*. (pp. 21–47). Hoboken, NJ: John Wiley & Sons.

Brilleslijper-Kater, S., & Baartman, H. (2000). What do young children know about sex? Research on sexual knowledge of children between the ages of 2 and 6 years. *Child Abuse Review, 9*(3),166–182.

Brilleslijper-Kater, S., Friedrich, W., & Corwin, D. (2004). Sexual knowledge and emotional reaction as indicators of sexual abuse in young children: Theory and research challenges. *Child Abuse & Neglect, 28,* 1007–1017.

Cavanagh-Johnson, T. (1993). Assessment of sexual behavior problems in preschool-aged and latency-aged children. *Sexual and Gender Identity Disorders, 2,* 431–449.

Cavanagh-Johnson, T., & Friend, C. (1995). Assessing young children's sexual behaviors in the context of sexual abuse evaluations. In T. Ney (Ed.), *True and false allegations of child sexual abuse: Assessment and case management* (pp. 49–72). New York: Brunner-Mazel Publishers.

Ceci, S., & Bruck, M. (1995). *Jeopardy in the courtroom*. Washington, DC: American Psychological Association.

Chaffin, M., Letourneau, E., & Silvosky, J. (2002). Adults, adolescents, and children who sexually abuse children: A developmental perspective. In J. Myers,

L. Berliner, J. Briere, C. Hendrix, C. Jenny, T. Reid, & T. Reid (Eds.), *The APSAC handbook on child maltreatment* (2nd ed., pp. 205–232). Thousand Oaks, CA: Sage Publications.

Corwin, D. (1988). Early diagnosis of child sexual abuse: Diminishing the lasting effects. In G. Wyatt & G. Powell (Eds.), *The lasting effects of child sexual abuse* (pp. 251–270). Newbury Park, CA: Sage.

Davies, S., Glaser, D., & Kossoff, R. (2000). Children's sexual play and behavior in pre-school settings: Staff's perceptions, reports, and responses. *Child Abuse & Neglect, 24*(10), 1329–1343.

Drach, K., Wientzen, J., & Ricci, L. (2001). The diagnostic utility of sexual behavior problems in diagnosing sexual abuse is a forensic child abuse evaluation clinic. *Child Abuse & Neglect, 25,* 489–503.

Dubowitz, H., Black, M., Harrington, D., & Verschoore, A. (1993). A follow up study of behavior problems associated with child sexual abuse. *Child Abuse & Neglect, 17,* 743–754.

Everson, M., & Boat, B. (1989). False allegations of sexual abuse by children and adolescents. *Journal of the American Academy of Child & Adolescent Psychiatry, 28*(2), 230–235.

Everson, M., & Sandoval, J. (2011). Forensic child sexual abuse evaluation: Assessing subjectivity and bias in professional judgments. *Child Abuse and Neglect, 35*(4), 287–297.

Faller, K. C. (2003). *Understanding and assessing child sexual maltreatment* (2nd ed.). Thousand Oaks, CA: Sage Publications.

Faller, K. C. (2007). *Interviewing children about sexual abuse: Controversies and best practice*. New York: Oxford University Press.

Faust, D., Bridges, A., & Ahern, D. (2009a). Methods for the identification of sexually abused children: Issues and needed features for abuse indicators. In K. Kuehnle & M. Connell (Eds.), *The evaluation of child sexual abuse allegations: A comprehensive guide to assessment and testimony* (pp. 3–19). Hoboken, NJ: John Wiley & Sons.

Faust, D., Bridges, A., & Ahern, D. (2009b). Methods for the identification of sexually abused children: Suggestions for clinical work and research. In K. Kuehnle & M. Connell (Eds.), *The evaluation of child sexual abuse allegations: A comprehensive guide to assessment and testimony* (pp. 49–66). Hoboken, NJ: John Wiley & Sons.

Finkelhor, D. (1994). Current information on the scope and nature of child sexual abuse. *The Future of Children, 4*(2), 31–53.

Finkelhor, D., & Browne, A. (1985). The traumatic impact of child sexual abuse: A conceptualization. *American Journal of Orthopsychiatry, 55*(4), 530–541.

Friedrich, W. N. (1993). Sexual victimization and sexual behavior in children: A review of recent literature. *Child Abuse & Neglect, 17,* 59–66.

Friedrich, W. N. (1995). The clinical use of the child sexual behavior inventory. *The APSAC Advisor, 8,* 1–20.

Friedrich, W. N. (1997). *Child sexual behavior inventory: Professional manual*. Odessa, FL: Psychological Assessment Resources.

Friedrich, W. N. (2002). *Psychological assessment of sexually abused children and their families*. Thousand Oaks, CA US: Sage Publications.

Friedrich, W. N. (2007). *Children with sexual behavior problems.* New York: W.W. Norton. Friedrich, W. N., Beilke, R. L., Urquiza, A. J. (1987). Children from sexually abusive families: A behavioral comparison. *Journal of Interpersonal Violence, 2,* 391–402.

Friedrich, W. N., Fisher, J., Broughton, D., Houston, M., & Shafran, C. (1998). Normative sexual behavior in children: A contemporary sample. *Pediatrics, 101,* 1–8.

Friedrich, W. N., Fisher, J., Dittner, C.A., Acton, Berliner, L., Butler, J., et al. (2001). Child sexual behavior inventory: Normative, psychiatric, and sexual abuse comparisons. *Child Maltreatment,* 6(1), 37–49.

Friedrich, W. N., Grambsch, P., Broughton, D., Kuiper, J., & Beilke, R. L. (1991). Normative sexual behavior in children. *Pediatrics, 88,* 456–464.

Friedrich, W. N., Grambsch, P., Damon, L., Hewitt, S., Koverola, C., Lang, R., et al. (1992). Child sexual behavior inventory: Normative and clinical samples. *Psychological Assessment, 4,* 303–311.

Friedrich, W. N., Olafson, E., & Faller, K. C. (2007). Standardized tests and measures. In K. Faller (Ed.), *Interviewing Children about Sexual Abuse: Controversies and Best Practice* (pp. 207–225). New York: Oxford University Press.

Friedrich, W. N., Trane, S., & Gully, K. (2005). It is a mistake to conclude that sexual abuse and sexualized behavior are not related: A reply to Drach, Wientzen, and Ricci (2001). *Child Abuse & Neglect, 29,* 297–302.

Gardner, R. (1987). *The parental alienation syndrome and the differentiation between fabricated and genuine child sexual abuse.* Cresskill, NJ: Creative Therapeutics.

Gardner, R. (1992). *True and false allegations of child sex abuse.* Cresskill, NJ: Creative Therapeutics.

Gelles, R. (1982). Applying research on family violence to clinical practice. *Journal of Marriage and the Family,* 44(1) 9–20.

Hall, D. K., Mathews, F., & Pearce, J. (1998). Factors associated with sexually behavior problems in young sexually abused children. *Child Abuse and Neglect, 22,* 1045–1063.

Herman, J. (1992). *Trauma and recovery.* New York: Basic Books.

Herman, S. (2009). Forensic child sexual abuse evaluations: Accuracy, ethics, and admissibility. In K. Kuehnle & M. Connell (Eds.), *The evaluation of child sexual abuse allegations: A comprehensive guide to assessment* (pp. 247–266). Hoboken, NJ: Wiley.

Hershkowitz, I., Orbach, Y., Lamb, M., Sternberg, K., & Horowitz, D. (2006). Dynamics of forensic interviews with suspected abuse victims who do not disclose abuse. *Child Abuse & Neglect,* 30(7), 753–769.

Hershkowitz, I., Orbach, Y., Sternberg, K., Pipe, M., Lamb, M., & Horowitz, D. (2007). Suspected victims of abuse who do not make allegations: An analysis of their interactions with forensic interviewers. *Child sexual abuse: Disclosure, delay, and denial* (pp. 97–113). Mahwah, NJ: Lawrence Erlbaum.

Jones, D. P. H., & McGraw, E. M. (1987). Reliable and fictitious accounts of sexual abuse to children. *Journal of Interpersonal Violence,* 2(1), 27–45.

Kendall-Tackett, K. E., Williams, L. M., & Finkelhor, D. (1993). The impact of sexual abuse on children: A review and synthesis of recent empirical studies. *Psychological Bulletin, 113,* 164–180.

Kuehnle, K. (1996). *Assessing allegations of child sexual abuse*. Sarasota, FL: Professional Resource Press.

Kuehnle, K. (1998). Child sexual abuse evaluations: The scientist-practitioner model. *Behavioral Sciences & the Law, 16*(1), 5–20.

Kuenhle, K., & Connell, M. (Eds.). (2009). *The evaluation of child sexual abuse allegations: A comprehensive guide to assessment and testimony*. Hoboken, NJ: John Wiley & Sons.

Lamb, M. E., Hershkowitz, I., Orbach, Y. & Esplin, P. W. (2008). *Tell me what happened. Structured investigative interviews of child victims and witnesses*. West Sussex, England: Wiley-Blackwell.

London, K., Bruck, M., Ceci, S. J., & Shuman, D. W. (2005). Disclosure of child sexual abuse: What does research tell us about the ways children tell? *Psychology, Public Policy, and Law, 11*, 194–224.

Lyon, T. D. (2007). False denials: Overcoming methodological biases in abuse disclosure research. In M.-E. Pipe, M. E. Lamb, Y. Orbach, & A. C. Cederborg (Eds.), *Child sexual abuse: Disclosure, delay and denial* (pp. 41–62). Mahwah, NJ: Lawrence Erlbaum.

Lyon, T. D., & Ahern, E. C. (2011). Disclosure of child sexual abuse. In J. Myers (Ed.), *The APSAC handbook on child maltreatment* (3d. ed., pp. 233–252). Newbury Park, CA: Sage.

Lyon, T. D., & Koehler, J. J. (1996). The relevance ratio: Evaluating the probative value of expert testimony in child sexual abuse cases. *Cornell Law Review, 82*, 43–78.

Merrill, L. L., Guimond, J. M., Thomsen, C. J., Milner, J. S. (2003). Child sexual abuse and number of sexual partners in young women: the role of abuse severity, coping style, and sexual functioning. *Journal of Consulting and Clinical Psychology, 71*(6), 987–996.

Paine, M. L., & Hansen, D. J. (2002). Factors influencing children to self-disclose sexual abuse. *Clinical Psychology Review, 22*, 271–295.

Ponterotto, J. G. (2005). Qualitative research in counseling psychology: A Primer on research paradigms and philosophy of science. *Journal of Counseling Psychology, 52*(2), 126–136.

Poole, D., & Lamb, M. (1998). *Investigative interviews of children*. Washington, DC: American Psychological Association.

Poole, D., & Lindsay, S. (1998). Assessing the accuracy of young children's reports: Lessons from the investigation of child sexual abuse. *Applied and Preventive Psychology, 7*(1), 1–26.

Poole, D. & Wolfe, M. (2009). Child development: Normative sexual and nonsexual behaviors that may be confused with symptoms of sexual abuse. In K. Kuehnle & M. Connell (Eds.), *The evaluation of child sexual abuse allegations: A comprehensive guide to assessment and testimony* (pp. 101–128). Hoboken, NJ: John Wiley & Sons.

Proeve, M. (2008). Issues in the application of Bayes' Theorem to child abuse decision-making. *Child Maltreatment, 14*, 114–120.

Sgroi, S., Porter, F., & Blick, L. (1982). Validation of sexual abuse. In S. Sgroi (Ed.), *Handbook of clinical intervention in child sexual abuse* (pp. 39–81). Lexington, MA: Lexington Books.

Tarren-Sweeney, M. (2008). Predictors of problematic sexual behavior among children with complex child maltreatment histories. *Child Maltreatment, 13*, 182–198.

Thornton, T. (2008). Does understanding individuals require idiographic judgment? *European Archives of Psychiatry and Clinica Neurosciences, 258*(5), 104–109.

Thornton, T. (2010). Narrative rather than idiographic approaches as counterpart to the nomothetic approach to assessment. *Psychopathology, 43*, 252–261.

Trocmé, N. & Bala, N. (2005). False allegations of abuse and neglect when parents separate. *Child Abuse & Neglect, 29*(11), 1333–1346.

Wells, R. D., McCann, J., Adams, J., Voris, J., & Ensign, J. (1995). Emotional, behavioral, and physical symptoms reported by parents of sexually abused, nonabused, and allegedly abused prepubescent females. *Child Abuse & Neglect, 19*, 155–163.

Wood, J. (1996). Weighing the evidence in sexual abuse evaluations: An introduction to Bayes's Theorem. *Child Maltreatment, 1*, 25–36.

AUTHOR NOTES

Mark D. Everson, PhD, is a professor of psychiatry and director of the Program on Childhood Trauma and Maltreatment at the University of North Carolina at Chapel Hill. He has served on the national board of directors of the American Professional Society on the Abuse of Children, and he co-chaired APSAC task forces that developed practice guidelines on investigative interviewing and on the use of anatomical dolls in cases of alleged child abuse. Dr. Everson's professional career has had a primary focus on improving forensic assessments of alleged child sexual abuse.

Kathleen Coulborn Faller, PhD, ACSW, DCSW, is a Marion Elizabeth Blue Professor of Children and Families in the School of Social Work at the University of Michigan and director of the Family Assessment Clinic, a program at the University of Michigan School of Social Work.

FUTURE DIRECTIONS

A Call for Field-Relevant Research about Child Forensic Interviewing for Child Protection

ERNA OLAFSON

University of Cincinnati College of Medicine; and Cincinnati Children's Hospital Medical Center, Cincinnati, Ohio, USA

This article reviews some sensitivity versus specificity imbalances in forensic investigations of child sexual abuse. It then proposes the development or further testing of additional approaches for those children who do not respond to the current, single-interview National Institute of Child Health and Human Development (NICHD) protocol. Although there are other interview protocols based on similar principles, the NICHD protocol has the strongest evidence base in both field and laboratory studies to elicit detailed and accurate information from children. Adaptations of the NICHD protocol or additional approaches need to be developed and tested for nondisclosing, partially disclosing, or recanting children, very young children, children with developmental disabilities, and children whose sexual abuse allegations are evaluated in the context of custody or visitation disputes.

INTRODUCTION: THE CHILDREN WE ARE MISSING

Absent from the chapter on forensic child sexual abuse evaluations by Steve Herman in the Kuehnle and Connell volume that is the focus of this special issue is a sense of urgency about intervening to rescue children who are being victimized by ongoing child sexual abuse or rape (Herman, 2009). Specificity is emphasized above sensitivity. It has been well established that physical evidence of child sexual abuse, even in cases of penetration, is rare (Frasier & Makoroff, 2006; Kellogg, Parra, & Menard, 1998). Other forms of hard corroborative evidence are available only in a minority of cases (Herman, 2009). Children's statements are often all we have to determine the facts of a case and, when necessary, to take action to protect children from ongoing sexual abuse. In this special issue, Lyon and colleagues argue for the probative value of children's statements. This paper supplements their work by proposing additional interview approaches. Because even Herman (2009) acknowledges that "hard" corroborative evidence is available in only a minority of cases, it is essential that those in child protection expand and improve child forensic interviewing so that children who have summoned the courage to disclose sexual abuse can be rescued rather than abandoned by the authorities to further sexual assault. This paper focuses primarily on child protection, so some of what is now known about the short- and long-term effects of sexual victimization on children and adult survivors will be briefly reviewed.

THE IMPACT OF CHILD SEXUAL ABUSE

Sexually abused children and adult survivors experience a range of psychiatric and behavioral problems, from minimal impacts to pervasive and disabling lifelong effects. Children who report more severe abuse (attempted or completed intercourse) are eight times more likely to experience depression than are nonabused children (Fergusson, Horwood, & Lynskey, 1996). Women with histories of childhood sexual abuse (CSA) are three to five times more likely to experience depression than nonabused women (Putnam, 2003). Children who have been sexually abused have higher rates of post-traumatic stress disorder than do those who have experienced other forms of maltreatment or trauma (Berliner, 2011; Dubner & Motta, 1999). In severe early childhood abuse cases of all kinds, brain development is affected so that both brain size and IQ are significantly reduced (Cohen, Perel, DeBellis, Friedman, & Putnam, 2002). Self-destructive behaviors, including drug dependence and alcoholism, are very strongly correlated with a history of CSA (Shin, Edwards, Heeren, & Amodeo, 2009). A history of CSA almost triples the risk for drug dependence in adult women (Kendler, et al., 2000). Sexual abuse alone increases the risk for adolescent drinking behavior almost as much as polyvictimization (Shin et al., 2009). The problematic sexual behaviors specific to CSA result in increased risk for HIV exposure, earlier pregnancies, revictimization, adult sexual offending, and prostitution (Andrews, Corry, Slade, & Issakids, & Swanston, 2004; Jesperson, Lalumiere, & Seto, 2009; Fargo, 2009; Noll, Shenk, & Putnam,

2009; Putnam, 2003; van Roode, Dickson, Herbison, & Paul, 2009; Widom & Ames, 1994).

As documented in a recent publication that reviews findings from a path-breaking 23-year longitudinal, multigenerational study about the impact of sexual abuse on female development, intrafamilial CSA has especially pervasive and severe negative sequelae (Trickett, Noll, & Putnam, 2011). The authors write that the "deleterious sequelae" to these sexual abuse victims occur across a "host of biopsychosocial domains," including earlier onsets of puberty, a wide range of psychiatric diagnoses, cognitive deficits, sexual revictimization, teen motherhood, and abuse and neglect of their own children (p. 453).

When CSA is not experienced by a young child as violent or painful, it still leaves a residue as the developing child learns that what came disguised as affectionate attention from a loving caregiver was instead sexual exploitation. The consequences can leave CSA survivors bewildered, avoidant, and profoundly distrustful about adult love and sexuality (Finkelhor & Browne, 1985). Childhood sexual victimization is also linked to intensely disabling feelings of shame that negatively affect the interpersonal relationships of victims well into adulthood (Feiring & Taska, 2005; Kim, Talbott, and Cicchetti. 2009).

The costs of child abuse are borne not only by victims and their families but also by society. A conservative estimate of direct and indirect costs of all forms of child abuse per year comes to $103.8 billion in 2007 dollars (Wang & Holton, 2007).

There are now evidence-based treatments for children and their caregivers to address the symptoms and behaviors associated with a history of child sexual abuse victimization and other childhood adversities (Cohen, Mannarino, & Deblinger, 2006; Deblinger & Heflin, 1996; Foa, Chrestman, & Gilboa-Schechtman, 2009), but children cannot be treated if the abuse is not discovered. In addition, some children rescued from CSA do well even without treatment if they have protective factors in their lives such as supportive nonoffending parents (Collishaw et al., 2007; DuMont, Widom, & Czaja, 2007; Jaffee, Caspi, Moffitt, Polo-Thomas, & Taylor, 2007).

FALSE POSITIVES OR FALSE NEGATIVES

In his chapter, Herman focuses on the danger of false positives, drawing on three papers from the 1990s that he states show that "hard corroborative evidence" is "quite common" in child sexual abuse cases (Herman, 2009, p. 258). Of the 677 cases examined in these three papers, Herman states that corroboration was available in 218, or just under one-third of cases (DiPietro, Runyan, & Frederickson, 1997; Dubowitz, Black, &

Harrington, 1992; Elliott & Briere, 1994). At 35% in the DiPietro and colleagues study and 37% in the Dubowitz and colleagues study, the "hard" corroborating evidence for CSA was limited to medical evidence. DiPietro and colleagues characterized their physical findings of 35% not as "hard" or "diagnostic" but as "suggestive of sexual abuse" (p. 138). The Dubowitz and colleagues medical findings were established before the extensive research of the 1990s altered much of the previous science about physical findings of CSA (Frasier & Makoroff, 2006). Current research shows that diagnostic medical evidence occurs in fewer than 10% of CSA cases (Frasier & Makoroff, 2006). In the third paper Herman cites, Elliott and Briere (1994) cited a lower corroborating evidence figure of 29.6%, which included not only medical evidence (16% of cases) but also offender confession, witnesses, and other evidence such as pornography. Herman fails to mention that in the Elliott and Briere sample, one-third of the children for whom external evidence of CSA existed either denied or recanted that they had been sexually abused, which, as Elliott and Briere pointed out, raises a troubling issue of "potential false negatives" (p. 275) during investigations.

Herman focuses, however, on false positives. He writes, "False positive error rates in forensic interviews are too high for these interviews to be used as the basis for making validity judgments about children's reports of CSA" (p. 261), and *"No legal decisions in child protection, civil, or criminal contexts should be based solely on an evaluators' judgment that an uncorroborated allegation of CSA is likely to be true"* (p. 261, italics in original). Because Lyon and colleagues critique Herman's arguments about false positives in another paper in this special issue, only the ethical issues Herman raises are covered here (refer to Everson, Sandoval, Berson, Crowson & Robinson, this issue, for a further rebuttal of Herman's criticisms of current forensic practice).

Eliminating child interviews as probative evidence would certainly solve the problem of false positives against adults wrongly accused of CSA, but it would do nothing to solve what may be the even greater problem of false negatives (Lyon, 1995, 2007). Adults will be safe. Children will not. If the child interview is only "soft" evidence on which no legal decisions can be based without hard corroboration, then many children who are being sexually abused and who try to disclose will not be protected from further abuse, their abusers will not be stopped, and other children may well be put at risk.

In a section on ethical implications, Herman appears to argue that evaluators are in greater danger of inflicting harm by substantiating false allegations than in failing to substantiate a true case, because, as he writes, "Ethically, if the available evidence is insufficient to substantiate a true abuse allegation, this is not the fault of the evaluator or investigators, assuming they made diligent, but unsuccessful, attempts to corroborate the allegation"

(p. 257). Herman argues that, by contrast, the evaluator is not the one who is harming the child by not substantiating because, "When a sexually abused child comes to the attention of the authorities, the major harm to that child has already been done, and this harm was caused by the perpetrator of the abuse" (p. 257). He does go on to argue, "Substantiating a true abuse allegation *may* [italics in original] protect the abused child from future abuse, prevent the perpetrator from abusing other children, and satisfy society's need to punish child molesters, however, it may do little to mitigate any harm that has already been caused to the child" (p. 257). One can debate the ethical issues about whether an evaluator inflicts harm when he or she fails to protect a child who has provided evidence of ongoing child sexual abuse when that evidence is limited to a full, detailed disclosure by that child given to an investigator in a well-done forensic interview. Even if Herman's estimates on corroborative evidence are accurate at one-third of all cases or 52% of those regarded as true (and, as argued, most current researchers find much lower rates of hard corroborative evidence), Herman's recommendations would leave half or two-thirds of children unprotected after they have been interviewed.

There is also an ethical issue about the failure to protect possible subsequent victims when true cases are not substantiated absent corroboration. Because many child molesters have more than one victim, with means for male-target victims reported at 150.2 and medians at 4.4 per perpetrator, other children may become targets when a disclosing child of actual child sexual abuse is not believed and action is not taken in the absence of corroborative evidence (Abel et al., 1987). Finally, Herman's statement that substantiating a true allegation "may do little to mitigate any harm that has been caused to the child" can be challenged. A well-established treatment for sexually abused children and their nonoffending caregivers is now available, with more than 15 studies (eight of them randomized controlled trials) establishing the effectiveness of this treatment (Trauma-Focused Cognitive Behavioral Therapy, or TFCBT) in "mitigating" the impact of child sexual victimization (Cohen, Deblinger, Mannarino, & Steer, 2004; Cohen et al., 2006; Deblinger & Heflin, 1996). Through the efforts of the federally funded National Child Traumatic Stress Network, mental health agencies throughout the United States have received or are receiving training in TFCBT, and a process to establish national certification for TFCBT providers is near completion. For therapists with a master's degree or above, a TFCBT training webinar is available at the Medical University of South Carolina website: http://tfcbt.musc.edu.

We should put at least as much energy and effort into avoiding false negatives (sensitivity) as false positives (specificity) in decisions about child sexual abuse allegations. Both cause harm. However, if, as the social psychological literature suggests, humans empathize more readily with others who resemble themselves (Dietz, Blackwell, Daley, & Bentley, 1982; Smith &

Firenze, 2003), it is possible that adults more readily feel the pain of the adult victim of a false positive than with the child victim of a false negative. A balanced perspective should focus equally on preventing both potentially tragic outcomes.

As Lyon and colleagues demonstrate in the article that appears in this issue, and as Herman acknowledges, we now have evidence-based principles to interview children and adolescents effectively, and these are best summarized in the various versions of the NICHD protocol by Michael Lamb and his colleagues, and in an abbreviated version by Thomas Lyon (Lamb, Hershkowitz, Orbach, & Esplin, 2008; Lyon, 2005). This paper calls for the development and study of additional approaches and protocols to reach those children not fully served by existing protocols. These may include very young children, children with developmental disabilities, children so traumatized or conflicted that they are unable or unwilling to disclose in the standard single-interview evaluations now most widely available, recanting children, and children for whom child sexual abuse allegations first arise in the context of parental separation with custody or visitation disputes. Emma, whose case vignette introduces this special issue, is a young child in a potential custody dispute whose safety and welfare may well have been better served if interviewers had other evidence-based interview methods available. The following recommendations for additional approaches or protocols apply to many children across these categories, and where they do not, this will be indicated.

FUTURE DIRECTIONS AND APPROACHES

The child forensic interviewing field has developed a solid scientific foundation in the past 15 years. Interviewers now have available one well-established, evidence-based child forensic interviewing approach, the National Institute of Child Health and Human Development (NICHD) protocol (Sternberg et al., 1997; Lamb et al., 2008; Kuehnle & Connell, 2009) that both Lyon and Herman endorse. However, the "rigid" adherence to the protocol that Herman recommends must be tempered by both Lamb's and Lyon's recognition that flexibility is essential and rigid adherence to scripted protocols will not reach every child. Both Lamb and Lyon suggest the development and testing of additional protocols and approaches to better interview the children such as Emma who do not respond to the NICHD protocol in its current form (Brown & Lamb, 2009; Lyon & Ahern, 2011). In addition, other interview methods that embody interviewing principles similar to those in the NICHD, such as John Yuille's Stepwise Interview, and the flexible guidelines taught at the National Child Advocacy Center, are still widely trained and used.

REPEATED INTERVIEWS AND EXTENDED INTERVIEW PROTOCOLS FOR RELUCTANT OR RECANTING CHILDREN

Everson and Faller call for a balanced perspective, so that not only are false allegations minimized, but also so that action can be taken to assist sexually abused children who have problems disclosing (see Everson and Faller, this issue). Brown and Lamb (2009) write, "Although the dangers of eliciting false reports from children have been discussed widely, little attention has been paid to an equally serious issue—children who have experienced abuse but do not disclose" (p. 309). Lamb and his colleagues (2008) mention the "motivational factors that make many children—more than a third of suspected victims and unknown numbers of children about whom no suspicions have been raised—reluctant to report abuse" (p. 17). Indeed, there exists consensus among researchers that many sexually abused children fail to disclose or tell only partially during a single interview (London, Bruck, Wright, & Ceci, 2008; Lyon, 2007). Statistics from Israel show that about a third of suspected victims do not disclose during interviews, in some cases perhaps because the child has not been abused, and in some cases perhaps because an abused child fails to disclose during the formal interview. A review of five years of Israeli cases (all interviewers in Israel use the NICHD protocol) revealed that children of all ages are less likely to disclose or allege abuse when the suspected perpetrator is a parent (Hershkowitz, Horowitz, & Lamb, 2005). Emma, the child in the introductory vignette, does not disclose in response to the NICHD protocol, but neither did the overwhelming majority in that Israeli study, which showed that girls aged three to six years old disclosed or alleged abuse in only 16.7% of cases when the allegation concerned a parent or parent figure and boys in only 12.3% of cases. A recent U.S. study found that that 18% of children did not disclose during formal interviews in cases where there was suspect confession (Pipe et al., 2007). Another U.S. study showed a recantation rate of 20% in dependency court cases where there was confirming medical evidence of child sexual abuse (Malloy, Lyon, & Quas, 2007).

Second interviews can also help partially disclosing children provide new details. In the only field study to date, Hershkowitz & Terner (2007) found that during a second interview using the NICHD protocol, children added 14% new details that were central to the allegations and 9% additional contextual details. Because this was a field study, the accuracy of information children provided in both interviews could not be independently assessed.

Are repeated interviews suggestive? La Rooy, Lamb, and Pipe (2009) reviewed the literature and concluded that repeated interviews are not in themselves suggestive, but they can "maximize the effects of suggestive interviewing" (p. 355), and that second interviews are more likely to provide accurate information when there are not long delays between interviews

(LaRooy & Lamb, 2008). However, clear guidelines need to be established for decisions about when to stop an interview with a reluctant child and when more than a single interview is appropriate (Hershkowitz et al., 2006).

Faller, Cordisco-Steele, and Nelson-Gardell (2010) summarize the current state of knowledge about repeated interviews or extended assessments as follows: "Research is needed to further clarify the criteria for extended assessments, more clearly articulate the number of sessions required, and define sequencing and techniques and strategies to be employed during an extended assessment" (p. 584). Brown and Lamb (2009) report that modifications to the NICHD protocol are now being developed and evaluated for reluctant children. To fully serve these children, protocols need to be developed and tested for repeated interviews (Faller et al., 2010). Updating and further research on the six-session National Child Advocacy Center extended forensic interview should also be considered (Carnes, Wilson, & Nelson-Gardell, 1999; Carnes, Nelson-Gardell, Wilson, & Orgassa, 2001). Finally, there is as yet no research about how best to interview children who have disclosed child sexual abuse and then recant (Lyon & Ahern, 2011).

DEVELOPMENTAL SCREENING

If developmental screening is necessary for investigative or forensic purposes (many courts want it done for preschoolers or those with developmental disabilities), there are no standardized, well-researched structured protocols for this screening. A brief scripted supplement for a standard protocol should be developed and tested for use when indicated, including guidelines for when and to whom (age ranges, developmental level) it should be administered.

INTERVIEW AIDS

The use of media aids in child forensic interviews remains a contested issue, and because of the mixed results to date, more research about the potential usefulness and suggestiveness of drawings and dolls should be undertaken, making use of optimal questioning strategies similar to those in the NICHD protocol rather than using the closed, leading, and misleading questions that have characterized much of the research to date (Pipe & Salmon, 2009).

The American Prosecutors Research Institute's *Finding Words* manual (Walters, Holmes, Bauer, & Vieth, 2003) provides guidelines for the use of anatomical dolls as demonstration aids following verbal disclosure; most other national trainings no longer include anatomical dolls as part of their basic forensic programs. The standard versions of the NICHD protocol contain no scripts for the use of media during interviews.

Although much of the early research focused on the dolls, researchers have studied drawings very extensively in the past decade, primarily in laboratory rather than field studies, with mixed results (Katz & Hershkowitz, 2010; Pipe & Salmon, 2009). Issues about whether and how to use anatomical drawings remain contested, with at least one major national training program still training interviewers in the Cornerhouse RATAC (rapport, anatomy identification, touch inquiry, abuse scenario, closure) protocol that routinely introduces anatomical drawings before the abuse inquiry so that the child can be asked to name body parts (Walters et al., 2003) and other experts cautioning against the use of anatomical drawings because of their potential suggestiveness (Lyon et al., current issue).

At least two recent field studies by researchers affiliated with the NICHD team offer a promising middle ground for use of the drawings to help children retrieve additional information about an event following disclosure (Aldridge et al., 2004; Katz & Hershkowitz, 2010). In their 2004 paper, Aldridge and colleagues published a structured protocol to use with a gender-neutral human figure drawing to elicit additional details to be used only after exhaustive questioning of children. They tested this approach on 90 4- to 13-year-old alleged child sexual abuse victims after NICHD verbal questioning had been completed. For all age groups, 18% of the total forensically relevant details obtained from children were obtained only when the drawing was used after full verbal questioning had been completed. The drawing was especially useful with the youngest children (aged 4 to 7), who gave 27% of the total details in the interview only with the drawing, contrasted with 12% of additional detail obtained from the 11- to 13-year-olds.

The authors caution that these additional details "came with a price" (p. 309). The drawings require use of more focused recognition prompts, and recognition rather than free recall prompts are generally associated with higher error rates from witnesses. In addition, because this was a field study, the accuracy of the information obtained could not be independently corroborated.

Katz's intriguing recent doctoral dissertation under the supervision of NICHD researcher Hershkowitz (Katz & Hershkowitz, 2010) deals with these recognition memory issues by having children create freehand drawings following full disclosure, followed by standard NICHD questioning while the child refers to the drawing. One hundred and twenty-five children aged 4 to 14 who had experienced single incidents of nonfamilial child sexual abuse were randomly assigned to drawing and no drawing groups. In the drawing group, after trained interviewers had exhaustively probed children's memories about the alleged event, they were given paper, a pencil, and an eraser and told to draw what happened. After 7 to 10 minutes, interviewers then said, "You've told me earlier what happened to you and now you've drawn it. The drawing is right here in front of you. Now please tell me everything that happened to you from the beginning to the end. You can also look at the drawing if you want" (pp. 173–174). Children in the nondrawing condition were also asked to tell everything a second time. In both conditions, the interviewers then continued to use NICHD sequential questioning strategy, focusing first on open questions and then moving gradually to more focused ones. Children in the drawing condition added 48% new information in response to open-ended prompts, whereas those in the nondrawing condition added 27% new information. In response to closed questions, children in both conditions added similar amounts of new information, which meant that the use of freehand drawings stimulated more additional detail from free recall than from recognition memory. This result is important because a generation of research has established the greater accuracy of children's free recall responses to open questions versus their recognition memory responses to more focused questions. Finally, even young children, whose pictures were often scribbled, provided large amounts of forensically relevant information after having made their drawings.

Because of these very promising results, it is hoped that further field research using freehand drawings on repeated events of child sexual abuse (as well as on other forms of childhood trauma and maltreatment) will produce results that can enhance children's witness capacity.

Children with Developmental Disabilities

It is well established that children and adults with disabilities experience higher rates of abuse than those without and that when questioned skillfully are capable of providing accurate information to investigators (Lamb et al, 2008). NICHD researchers have developed and are field testing a version of the protocol to interview both adults and children with developmental disabilities (Lamb et al., 2008). Changes include a longer rapport-building phase, provision of more interviewer support throughout the interview, shorter and simpler questions, a slower pace, and more frequent use of second interviews.

Additional Protocols

Lamb and colleagues have called for research on narrative elaboration and cognitive interviewing in the field, especially with children who have a history of trauma (Brown & Lamb, 2009). Because disclosures adequate for protection are especially challenging with young children (and even more so for the purposes of prosecution), adding narrative elaboration techniques to the interviewer toolkit for either single or extended interview protocols may increase the number of children protected during the crucial early years until about age seven when the brain and nervous system are developing and ongoing child sexual abuse can be especially damaging (Putnam, 2006). For older children and for adults, the cognitive interview has a robust evidence base and shows promise for children of school age and older in helping them report additional information. Field research on the cognitive interview is still needed with children interviewed after long delays between event and investigation and about traumatic events (Brown & Lamb, 2009).

Narrative elaboration is not a complete interview protocol but it could well be incorporated into standard protocols, when preschoolers or those with developmental delays are being interviewed. The narrative elaboration technique (NET) provides pre-interview training by using pictures to cue information retrieval. One advantage of these cue cards is that they limit the kinds of questions interviewers ask to those that young children or those with developmental delays can answer; the cue cards focus on "who, where, what happened, what was said, what was felt" and avoid the more difficult questions about "when, why, how long, how many times." Children are first trained to talk about neutral experiences using the cards and are then questioned about the topic of concern using the cards again (Saywitz & Snyder, 1993, 1996). In laboratory studies, NET helps children with mental retardation and preschoolers report events more completely, with no increase in errors or reports of false events (Camparo, Wagner, & Saywitz, 2001). NET is also effective for older children (aged eight to nine) with long delays after an event (Brown & Pipe, 2003). The NET still needs to be researched in field studies of actual abuse and criminal allegations. Brown and Lamb (2009) write that the full NET or components of it may help children of all ages, including those with cognitive delays, "report more forensically relevant details about experienced events" but add that further research is needed (p. 304).

The five-stage cognitive interview (CI) was developed for adult witnesses by Fisher and Geiselman (1992) and subsequently adapted for children by Saywitz and others (Fisher & Geiselman, 1992; Saywitz, Geiselman, & Bornstein, 1992). Some studies have included children as young as four. The CI probed recall component could be incorporated into standard protocols such as the NICHD after open questioning has invited a full, but not sufficiently detailed, disclosure (Brown & Lamb, 2009). Probed recall (cognitive reinstatement) contains mnemonic techniques to aid retrieval of information from memory. After adult witnesses have reported everything they can remember using free recall in response to open questions, they are guided in context reinstatement by picturing themselves at the place of the event and asked what they saw, smelled, heard, felt, tasted, thought, and then who was there, and what was said. They are then asked to describe the event completely again from the beginning to the end, then from the end to the beginning, and finally from a different perspective, such as that of another person who was also present.

Adaptations must be made for children. Children as young as seven can do the reverse order with supportive scaffolding provided by the interviewer. It is generally agreed that imagining the event from another perspective is not recommended for forensic interviews with any child or adolescent witness because it departs from real reporting about real events. Finally, because of the potential suggestiveness of cognitive reinstatement, the probed recall portion of the CI should not be used to elicit a disclosure from children or adolescents but only to trigger recall of greater detail post disclosure after free recall has been exhausted.

In many laboratory studies with adult witnesses, the CI significantly increases the amount of information reported, with no decrease in accuracy. Results with children have been mixed but generally positive, with improved recall and increased resistance to suggestion or with an increased, but still proportional, number of errors (Brown & Lamb, 2009).

INTERVIEWER MANNER

The NICHD protocol is used universally in Israel. An enormous archive is available there on audiotape, but because it has been studied primarily through the use of transcripts of audiotaped interviews, the research supporting it has not evaluated how facial expressions, bodily posture, and other nonverbal interviewer behaviors could affect children's responsiveness. Researchers have established that young children report more on free recall and are less suggestible when interviewers are warm and friendly rather than cold, authoritarian, or condescending (Bottoms, Quas, & Davis, 2007; Davis & Bottoms, 2002). A future research project for laboratory and field research on videotaped interviews using the NICHD protocol and adding coding for interviewer manner could be informative.

PEER REVIEW AND SUPERVISION

Even those children who respond to the NICHD protocol will not be interviewed competently if trained interviewers do not implement it well. Ingoing fidelity to this protocol is achieved only with regular support. It has now been shown that interviewers trained in the NICHD protocol fail to fully implement its questioning strategies unless there is ongoing peer review and supervision. In one U.S. study, even after six months of supervision, interviewers returned to more closed questions and asked them earlier in interviews after peer review ended (Lamb, Sternberg, Orbach, Esplin, & Mitchell, 2002). Most American jurisdictions, even those that use the NICHD protocol, have not established the ongoing supervision and peer review that is necessary to maintain evidence-based interviewing (Brown & Lamb, 2009;

Herman, 2009). Israel has established and still maintains bimonthly peer review/supervision for child forensic interviewers. Perhaps a delegation of U.S. experts should visit them to study how this has been achieved, funded, and maintained.

CHILD SEXUAL ABUSE ALLEGATIONS IN THE CONTEXT OF CUSTODY DISPUTES

Child sexual abuse allegations in the context of custody disputes are not directly addressed in the 2009 Kuehnle and Connell book, but the family court is a legal arena in which child protection through adequate evaluation is essential, whereas evidence-based child interviewing protocols are relatively uncommon, and many abused children may be missed.

In the United States, most divorcing couples with minor children settle their cases without custody disputes so that only about 10% dispute custody in the courts. In Canada as well, "Most parents who separate resolve disputes about their children without going to court" (Bala & Schuman, 1999, p. 195).

We lack current national research data for the United States about how custody-disputing families differ from the great majority of families who settle out of court. Are custody disputes mere gambits in the divorce wars, or do they arise because many parents who contest custody are motivated by genuine concerns about children's safety? Older U.S. research about false allegations of child sexual abuse in contested custody cases nationwide found that in the tiny minority of custody access cases where child sexual abuse allegations arose, 14% were believed to be false (Thoennes & Tjaden, 1990). As with subsequent studies in Australia and Canada, the U.S. researchers also found that children and families were badly served because the family courts, child protection system, and the dependency courts were poorly coordinated.

Australian researchers reviewed court records of 200 randomly selected families in which child abuse allegations were made in the Family Court of Australia in custody access cases (Brown, Frederico, Hewitt, & Sheehan, 2000, 2001). Although neglect is the most common form of child maltreatment reported to the authorities in Australia, the most common forms of child abuse found in these custody access cases were sexual and/or physical abuse (70%). Much of this abuse was severe. There were also high rates of substance abuse and partner violence. Only 22.5% of these abuse cases were previously known to the child protection authorities, and 70% of the cases were substantiated. It is significant that false cases appeared to be no more common than in noncustody or access circumstances; 9% of the custody-disputing cases were found to be false, which is the same incidence found in the general Australian child protection system. The authors conclude that this research "indicates that child abuse within de facto and legal marriage breakdown is real, that it is abuse of a serious kind, that child abuse is a major aspect of family courts' workload, [and] that family courts do not deal well with the children, but that they can improve" (Brown et al., 2001, p. 858). The Family Court of Australia has now established Project Magellan to improve coordination among the various systems that serve custody disputing families where there are abuse allegations (Brown, 2002).

Trocme and Bala (2005) examined a representative sample of child maltreatment cases in a national Canadian study and compared those that involved custody or access disputes with those that did not. They used the clinical judgment made by the investigating child welfare worker and found that rates of intentionally false allegations were higher in the custody or access subsample (12%) than in the total sample (4%). They also found that intentionally false allegations of neglect were far more common than intentionally false allegations of abuse, and noncustodial parents (mostly fathers) were far more likely to make intentionally false allegations (43% of false allegations) than were custodial parents (mostly mothers, 14%). However, for child sexual abuse, custodial parents were the source of 19% of the false reports of child sexual abuse and noncustodial parents 16%, with neighbors, relatives, and others responsible for the remaining false CSA reports. The authors note that a limitation of the study is that the determination of falseness was made by the investigating child welfare workers, which at least one U.S. study has shown may approach these cases with a nonsubstantiation bias (McGraw & Smith, 1992).

Regional U.S. studies add useful, if partial information. In Elliott's and Briere's (1994) examination of 399 children aged 8–15 at a single sexual abuse evaluation center in California, they found no higher rates of false allegations when custody was disputed. Faller and DeVoe (1995) examined a sample of 215 cases of child sexual abuse allegations during divorce in a single Midwestern university-based clinic. Of the 45 false or possibly false cases, the clinic classified 10, or 4.7%, as "knowingly made false allegations" (p. 9). In cases where Faller's Michigan clinic coded child sexual abuse as "likely," the domestic relations court made rulings for no contact or supervised visitation in 60.3% of cases, but 37.2% of children were left with unprotected contact with the alleged CSA perpetrator in the cases the clinic had coded as "likely." Those cases in which the allegation came from the mother rather than from other sources were less likely to result in protection of the child from the accused.

Because so much previous literature has focused on higher rates of false allegations in the context of custody disputes, it is worth asking whether there might also be higher rates of true allegations in this context. Faller and Devoe (1995) have identified three reasons why this may be so: "The breakup of a marriage may be the precipitator of disclosure of child sexual abuse, and marital disruption may increase risk for sexual abuse. . ." or "parents may choose to divorce when they discover sexual abuse" (p. 20). In addition, single-parent households in the immediate aftermath of parental separation can be chaotic, high risk environments in which parental supervision may be compromised, and the children may be exposed to and left unsupervised with numerous other people including new sexual partners of the parents (Wallerstein & Kelly, 1980).

As Brown and colleagues (2000, 2001) suggest for Australia and Faller shows for Michigan, family courts are not always doing an adequate job in protecting children in these high-risk cases. The "best interests of the child" standard should include systematic risk assessment protocols. If family courts have a central role in child protection, then their investigators need training in evidence-based interview methods designed to elicit full and accurate information from children at potential risk. But, as Faller (2000) has noted, "Personnel in the social service and legal systems that address situations of divorce usually have no particular expertise in investigating child maltreatment" (p. 16).

The situation could be remedied with development and research of a structured protocol for custody evaluators, using established NICHD principles and including standard risk and safety assessment questions. Much of this work has already been accomplished by Karen Saywitz and her colleagues (Saywitz, Camparo, & Romanoff, 2010), who outline 10 principles to interview children in custody cases, drawing heavily on the NICHD research but omitting questions about safety or risk. These principles could be reformatted into a structured protocol, risk assessment questions incorporated, and training programs established to improve practice nationwide in social service and legal systems that deal with custody and access disputes.

Children may be at heightened safety risks for all forms of child maltreatment, including child sexual abuse, following parental separation, so that systematic risk assessment screening as a standard part of child custody evaluations should be considered. "No fault" does not guarantee "no risk." The focus on the possibility of false allegations or parental alienation in custody and access disputes (Bernet et al., 2008), a focus that has often included an implicit antimother bias, can obscure what may well be the more common problem of heightened risk for child maltreatment in the context of separated parents. Research results about the rate of deliberately false allegations of child sexual abuse in custody and access disputes is mixed, but no study finds that rates are very high.

CONCLUSION

Because unrecognized and untreated child sexual abuse constitutes a major public health problem, it is essential to expand the range of interviewing methods to reach those children not yet fully served by the single fully evidence-based protocol. NICHD protocol developers recognize this challenge and are working to expand the protocol to better interview reluctant children and developmentally delayed children. This paper recommends protocol development and testing for very young preschoolers, for children with developmental disabilities, for reluctant children or those who recant, and for children interviewed in the context of custody and visitation disputes. There is also a need for improved, standardized and fully funded peer review structures for agencies, child advocacy centers, and police departments who conduct the majority of child forensic interviews in the United States so that evidence-based principles are implemented with fidelity. Finally, family and domestic relations courts must expand the training for custody evaluators to incorporate principles already well established to assess for risk or maltreatment.

REFERENCES

Abel, G. G., Becker, J. V., Mittelman, M., Cunningham-Rathner, J., Rouleau, J. L., Murphy, W. D. (1987). Self-reported sex crimes of nonincarcerated paraphiliacs. *Journal of Interpersonal Violence, 2*(1), 3–25.

Aldridge, J., Lamb, M., Sternberg, K., Orbach, Y., Esplin, P., & Bowler, L. (2004). Using a human figure drawing to elicit information from alleged sexual abuse victims. *Journal of Consulting and Clinical Psychology, 72*(2), 304–316.

Andrews, G., Corry, J., Slade, T., Issakids, C., & Swanston, H. (2004). Child sexual abuse. In M. Essati, A. D. Lopez, A. Rodgers, & C. J. I. Murray (Eds.), *Comparative quantification of health risks: Global and regional burden of disease attributable to major risk factors* (pp. 1851–1940). Geneva: World Health Organization.

Bala, N., & Schuman, J. (1999). Allegations of sexual abuse when parents have separated. *Canadian Family Law Quarterly, 17*, 191–241.

Berliner, L. (2011). Child sexual abuse: Definitions, prevalence, and consequences. In J. E. B. Myers (Ed.), *The APSAC handbook on child maltreatment* (3rd ed.; pp. 215–232. Los Angeles: Sage.

Bernet, W., Boch-Galhau, W. V., Kenan, J., Kinlan, J., Lorandos, D., Sauber, R., et al. (2008). Parental alienation disorder and DSM-V. *Disorders in Childhood and Adolescence Work Group for the Diagnostic and Statistical Manual of Mental Disorders,* Fifth. Unpublished manuscript.

Bottoms, B. B., Quas, J. A., & Davis, S. A. (2007). The influence of interviewer-provided social support on children's suggestibility, memory, and disclosures. In M. E. Pipe, M. E. Lamb, Y. Orbach, & A. C. Cederborg (Eds.), *Child sexual abuse: Disclosure, delay, and denial* (pp. 135–157). Mahwah, NJ: Erlbaum.

Brown, T. (2002). Magellan's discoveries: An evaluation of a program for managing family court parenting disputes involving child abuse allegations. *Family Court Review, 40*(3), 320–328.

Brown, T., Frederico, M., Hewitt, L., & Sheehan, R. (2000). Revealing the existence of child abuse in the context of marital breakdown and custody and access disputes. *Child Abuse and Neglect, 24*(6), 849–859.

Brown, T., Frederico, M., Hewitt, L., & Sheehan, R. (2001). The child abuse and divorce myth. *Child Abuse Review*, *10*(2), 113–124.

Brown, D., & Lamb, M. E. (2009). Forensic interviews with children. In K. Kuehnle & M. Connell (Eds.), *The evaluation of child sexual abuse allegations* (pp. 299–325). Hudson, NJ: Wiley.

Brown, D. A., & Pipe, M. E. (2003). Variations on a technique: Enhancing children's recall using narrative elaboration training. *Applied Cognitive Psychology*, *17*, 377–399.

Camparo, L. B., Wagner, J. T., & Saywitz, K. J., (2001). Interviewing children about real and fictitious events: Revisiting the narrative elaboration procedure. *Law and Human Behavior*, *25*, 63–80.

Carnes, C. N., Nelson-Gardell, D., Wilson, C., & Orgassa, U. C. (2001). Extended forensic evaluation when sexual abuse is suspected: A multi-site field study. *Child Maltreatment*, *6*, 230 242.

Carnes, C. N., Wilson, C., & Nelson-Gardell, D. (1999). Extended forensic evaluation when sexual abuse is suspected. A model and preliminary data. *Child Maltreatment*, *4*, 242–254.

Cohen, J. A., Deblinger, E., Mannarino, A. P., & Steer, R. A., (2004). A multisite, randomized controlled clinical trial for children with sexual abuse-related PTSD symptoms. *Journal of American Academy of Child and Adolescent Psychiatry*, *43*, 393–402.

Cohen, J. A., Mannarino, A. P., & Deblinger, E. (2006). *Treating trauma and traumatic grief in children and adolescents*. New York: The Guilford Press.

Cohen, J. A., Perel, J. M., DeBellis, M. D., Friedman, J. J., & Putnam, F. W. (2002). Treating traumatized children: Clinical implications of the psychobiology of posttraumatic stress disorder. *Trauma, Violence & Abuse*, *3*, 91–108.

Collishaw, S., Pickles, A., Messer, J., Rutter, M., Shearer, C., & Maughan, B. (2007). Resilience to adult psychopathology following childhood maltreatment: Evidence from a community sample. *Child Abuse & Neglect*, *31*(3), 211–229.

Davis, L., & Bottoms, B. L. (2002). Effects of social support on children's eyewitness reports: A test of the underlying mechanism. *Law and human behavior*, *26*, 185–215.

Deblinger, E., & Heflin, A. H. (1996). *Treating sexually abused children and their nonoffending parents: A cognitive behavioral approach*. Thousand Oaks, CA: Sage.

Dietz, S. R., Blackwell, K. T., Daley, P. C., & Bentley, B. J. (1982). Measurement of empathy toward rape victims and rapists. *Journal of Personality and Social Psychology*, *43*, 372–384.

DiPietro, E. K., Runyan, D. K., & Fredrickson, D. D. (1997). Predictors of disclosure during medical evaluation for suspected sexual abuse. *Journal of Child Sexual Abuse*, *6*(1), 133–142.

Dubner, A. E., & Motta, R. W. (1999). Sexually and physically abused foster care children and posttraumatic stress disorder. *Journal of Consulting and Clinical Psychology*, *67*, 367–373.

Dubowitz, H., Black, M., & Harrington, D. (1992). The diagnosis of child sexual abuse. *American Journal of Diseases of Children*, *146*(6), 688–693.

DuMont, K. A., Widom, C. S., & Czaja, S. J. (2007). Predictors of resilience in abuse and neglected children grown-up: The role of individual and neighborhood characteristics. *Child Abuse & Neglect, 31*(3), 255–274.

Elliott, D., & Briere, J. (1994). Evaluations of older children: Disclosures and symptomatology. *Behavioral Sciences and the Law, 12*(3), 261–277.

Faller, K. C. (2000). Child abuse and divorce: Competing priorities and agendas and practical suggestions. *Journal of Aggression, Trauma, & Maltreatment, 2*(4), 167–196.

Faller, K. C., Cordisco-Steele, L., & Nelson-Gardell, D. (2010). Allegations of sexual abuse of a child: What to do when a single forensic interview isn't enough. *Journal of Child Sexual Abuse, 19,* 572–589.

Faller, K. C., & DeVoe, E. (1995). Allegations of sexual abuse in divorce. *Journal of Child Sexual Abuse, 4*(4), 1–25.

Fargo, J. D. (2009). Pathways to adult sexual revictimization: Direct and indirect behavioral risk factors across the lifespan. *Journal of Interpersonal Violence, 24,* 1771–1791.

Feiring, C., & Taska, L. S. (2005). The persistence of shame following sexual abuse: A longitudinal look at risk and recovery. *Child Maltreatment, 10,* 337–349.

Fergusson, D., Horwood, L., & Linskey, M. (1996). Childhood sexual abuse and psychiatric disorder in young adulthood, II: Psychiatric outcomes of childhood sexual abuse. *Journal of the Academy of Child and Adolescent Psychiatry, 35,* 1365–1374.

Finkelhor, D., & Browne, A. (1985). The traumatic impact of child sexual abuse: A conceptualization. *Journal of Orthopsychiatry, 55*(4), 530–541.

Fisher, R. P., & Geiselman, R. E., (1992). *Memory-enhancing techniques for investigating interviewing: The cognitive interview.* Springfield, IL: Charles C Thomas.

Foa, E. B., Chrestman, K. R., & Gilboa-Schechtman, E. (2009). *Prolonged exposure therapy for adolescents with PTSD: Emotional processing of traumatic experiences.* Oxford, England: Oxford University Press.

Frasier, L. D., & Makoroff, K. L. (2006). Medical evidence and expert testimony in child sexual abuse. *Juvenile and Family Court Journal, 57,* 41–50.

Herman, S. (2009). Forensic child sexual abuse evaluations: Accuracy, ethics, and admissibility. In K. Keuhnle & M. Connell (Eds.), *The evaluation of child sexual abuse allegations.* Hoboken, NJ: John Wiley & Sons.

Hershkowitz, I., Horowitz, D., Lamb, M. (2005). Trends in children's disclosure of abuse in Israel: A national study. *Child Abuse & Neglect, 29,* 1203–1214.

Hershkowitz, I., Orbach, Y., Lamb, M. E., Pipe, M. E., Sternberg, K. J., & Horowitz, D. (2006). Dynamics of forensic interviews with suspected abuse victims who do not disclose abuse. *Child Abuse and Neglect, 30,* 753–769.

Hershkowitz, I, & Terner, A. (2007). The effects of repeated interviewing on children's forensic statements of sexual abuse. *Applied Cognitive Psychology, 21,* 1131–1143.

Jaffee, S. R., Caspi, A., Moffitt, T. E., Polo-Thomas, M., & Taylor, A. (2007). Individual, family, and neighborhood factors distinguish resilient from non-resilient maltreated children: A cumulative stressors model. *Child Abuse & Neglect, 31*(3), 231–253.

Jespersen, A. F., Lalumiere, M. L., & Seto, M. C. (2009). Sexual abuse history among adult sex offenders and non-sex offenders: A meta-analysis. *Child Abuse and Neglect, 33,* 179–192.

Katz, C., & Hershkowitz, I. (2010). The effects of drawing on children's accounts of sexual abuse. *Child Maltreatment, 15*(2), 171–179.

Kim, J., Talbott, N. L., & Cicchetti, D. (2009). Childhood abuse and current interpersonal conflict: The role of shame. *Child Abuse and Neglect, 33,* 362–371.

Kellogg, N. D., Parra, J. M., & Menard, S. (1998, July). Children with anogenital symptoms and signs referred for sexual abuse evaluations. *Archives of Pediatrics and Adolescent Medicine, 152*(7), 634–641.

Kendler, K. S., Bulik, C. M., Silberg, J., Hettema, J. M., Myers, M. S., & Prescott, C. A. (2000). Childhood sexual abuse and adult psychiatric and substance use disorders in women. *Archives of General Psychiatry, 57,* 953–959.

Kuehnle, K., & Connell, M. (Eds.). (2009). *The evaluation of child sexual abuse allegations* (1st ed.). Hoboken: John Wiley & Sons.

Lamb, M. E., Hershkowitz, I., Orbach, Y., & Esplin, P. W. (2008). *Tell me what happened: Structured investigative interviews of child victims and witnesses.* West Sussex, England: Wiley-Blackwell.

Lamb, M. E., Sternberg, K. J., Orbach, Y., Esplin, P. W., & Mitchell, S. (2002). Is ongoing feedback necessary to maintain the quality of investigative interviews with allegedly abused children? *Applied Developmental Science, 6,* 35–41.

La Rooy, D., & Lamb, M. (2008). What happens when young witnesses are interviewed more than once. *Forensic Update.* Retrieved from http://www.larooy.net/FU.pdf

La Rooy, D., Lamb, M., & Pipe, M. E. (2009). Repeated interviewing: A critical evaluation of the risks and potential benefits. In K. Kuehnle & M. Connell (Eds.), *Child sexual abuse: Research, evaluation, and testimony for the courts* (pp. 327–364). Hoboken, NJ: John Wiley.

London, K., Bruck, M., Wright, D., & Ceci, S. (2008). Review of the contemporary literature on how children report sexual abuse to others: Findings, methodological issues, and implication for forensic interviewers. *Memory, Special Issues: New Insights into Trauma and Memory, 16,* 29–47.

Lyon, T. D. (1995). False allegations and false denials in child sexual abuse. *Psychology, Public Policy, and Law, 1*(2), 429–437.

Lyon, T. D. (2005). *Ten-step investigative interview.* Retrieved from http://works.bepress.com/thomaslyon/5/

Lyon, T. D. (2007). False denials: Overcoming methodological biases in abuse disclosure research. In M. E. Pipe, M. E. Lamb, Y. Orbach, & A. C. Cederborg (Eds.), *Child sexual abuse: Disclosure, delay, and denial* (pp. 41–62). Mahwah, NJ: Erlbaum.

Lyon, T. D., & Ahern, E. C. (2011). Disclosure of child sexual abuse. In J. E. B. Myers (Ed.), *The APSAC handbook on child maltreatment.* Thousand Oaks, CA: Sage Publications.

Malloy, L. C., Lyon, T. D., & Quas, J. A. (2007). Filial dependency and recantation in child sexual abuse allegations. *Journal of the American Academy of Child and Adolescent Psychiatry, 46,* 162–170.

McGraw, J. M., & Smith, H. A. (1992). Child sexual abuse allegations amidst divorce and custody proceedings: Refining the validation process. *Journal of Child Sexual Abuse, 1*(1), 49–62.

Noll, J. G., Shenk, C. E., & Putnam, F. W. (2009). Childhood sexual abuse and adolescent pregnancy: A meta-analytic update. *Journal of Pediatric Psychology, 34*, 366–378.

Pipe, M. E., Lamb, M. E., Orbach, O., Stewart, H. L., Sternberg, K. J., & Esplin, P. W. (2007). Factors associated with non-disclosure of suspected abuse during forensic interviews. In M. E. Pipe, M. E. Lamb, Y. Orbach, & A. C. Cederborg (Eds.) *Child sexual abuse: Disclosure, delay, and denial* (pp. 77–96). Mahwah, NJ: Erlbaum.

Pipe, M. E., & Salmon, K. (2009). Dolls, drawing, body diagrams, and other props: Role of props in investigative interviews. In K. Kuehnle & M. Connell (Eds.), *The evaluation of child sexual abuse allegations: A comprehensive guide to assessment and testimony.* Hoboken, NJ: John Wiley & Sons.

Putnam, F. W. (2003). Ten-year research update review: Child sexual abuse. *Journal of the American Academy of Child and Adolescent Psychiatry, 42*(3), 269–278.

Putnam, F. W. (2006). The impact of trauma on child development. *Juvenile and Family Court Journal, 57*(1), 1–12.

Saywitz, K., Camparo, L. B., & Romanoff, A. (2010). Interviewing children in custody cases: Implications of research and policy for practice. *Behavioral Sciences and the Law, 28*, 542–562.

Saywitz, K. J., Geiselman, R. E., & Bornstein, G. K. (1992). Effects of cognitive interviewing and practice on children's recall performance. *Journal of Applied Psychology, 77*, 744–756.

Saywitz, K. J., & Snyder, L., (1993). Improving children's testimony with preparation. In G. S. Goodman & B. L. Bottoms (Eds.), *Child victims, child witnesses: Understanding and improving testimony* (pp. 117–146). New York: Guilford.

Saywitz, K. J., & Snyder, L. (1996). Narrative elaboration: Test of a new procedure for interviewing children. *Journal of Consulting & Clinical Psychology, 64*, 1347–1357.

Shin, U. H., Edwards, E., Heeren, T., & Amodeo, M. (2009). Relationship between multiple forms of maltreatment by a parent or guardian and adolescent alcohol use. *The American Journal of Addiction, 18*, 226–234.

Smith, C. A., & Firenze, I. H. (2003). Examining rape empathy from the perspective of the victim and the assailant. *Journal of Applied Social Psychology, 33*(3), 476–498.

Sternberg, K. J., Lamb, M. E., Hershkowitz, I., Yudilevitch, L., Orbach, Y., Esplin, P. W., et al. (1997). Effects of introductory style on children's abilities to describe experiences of sexual abuse. *Child Abuse and Neglect, 21*, 1133–1146.

Thoennes, N., & Tjaden, P. (1990). The extent, nature, and validity of sexual abuse allegations in custody/visitation disputes. *Child Abuse and Neglect, 14*, 151–163.

Trickett, P. K., Noll, J. G., Putnam, F. W. (2011). The impact of sexual abuse on female development: Lessons from a multigenerational, longitudinal research study. *Development and Psychopathology, 23*(2), 453–476.

Trocmé, N., & Bala, N. (2005). False allegations of abuse when parents separate: Canadian Incidence Study of Reported Child Abuse and Neglect, 1998. *Child Abuse & Neglect, 29*(12), 1333–1345.

Van Roode, T., Dickson, N., Herbison, P., & Paul, C. (2009). Child sexual abuse and persistence of risky sexual behavior and negative sexual outcomes over adulthood: Findings from a birth cohort. *Child Abuse and Neglect, 33*, 161–172.

Wallerstein, J. S., & Kelly, J. B. (1980). *Surviving the breakup: How children and parents cope with divorce.* New York: Basic Books.

Walters, S., Holmes, L., Bauer, G., & Vieth, V. (2003). *Finding words: Half a nation by 2010 interviewing children and preparing for court.* Alexandria, VA: American Prosecutors Research Institute.

Wang, C. T., & Holton, J. (2007). Total estimated cost of child abuse in the United States. In *Economic impact study.* Chicago: Prevent Child Abuse America.

Widom, C. S., & Ames, M. A. (1994). Criminal consequences of childhood sexual victimization. *Child Abuse & Neglect, 18*, 303–318.

AUTHOR NOTE

Erna Olafson, PhD, PsyD, is associate professor of clinical psychiatry and pediatrics at Cincinnati Children's Hospital Medical Center and the University of Cincinnati College of Medicine. She has directed the Cincinnati Children's Hospital Childhood Trust Child Forensic Training Program since 1999.

# Section 2:

Commentaries and Responses

"Nobody's Perfect"—Partial Disagreement with Herman, Faust, Bridges, and Ahern

JOHN E. B. MYERS

University of the Pacific, Sacramento, California, USA

This article takes issue with aspects of chapters in Kathryn Kuehnle and Mary Connell's 2009 book, The Evaluation of Child Abuse Allegations: A Comprehensive Guide to Assessment and Testimony.

Determining whether a child was sexually abused is a tremendous clinical and legal challenge. The U.S. Supreme Court noted this difficulty in *Pennsylvania v. Ritchie* (1987) in which the Court wrote, "Child abuse is one of the most difficult crimes to detect and prosecute, in large part because there often are no witnesses except the victim" (p. 60). In a similar vein, the New York Court of Appeals wrote in *In re Nicole V.* (1987), "Abuse is difficult to detect because the acts are predominantly nonviolent and usually occur in secret rendering the child the only witness" (p. 915).

In litigation, abuse is established—proven—with evidence.[1] Evidence includes testimony from witnesses, hearsay statements,[2] documents, and physical evidence such as semen, genital injury, and fingerprints. There are two types of witnesses: lay witnesses (sometimes called percipient witnesses) and expert witnesses. In sexual abuse litigation, expert testimony is provided by medical and mental health professionals. Whereas physicians and nurses describe physical evidence of abuse, mental health professionals describe psychological evidence of abuse. Both types of expert testimony are complicated and, to varying degrees, controversial. The most controversial mental health testimony is testimony that a particular child was sexually abused or has symptoms "consistent with" sexual abuse (Melton & Limber, 1989; Melton, Petrila, Poythress, & Slobogin, 2007; Myers, 2010). A review of court cases indicates occasional use of dubious mental health testimony that a child was abused or has symptoms consistent with abuse (See Myers, 2011).

Mental health testimony offered to prove sexual abuse is complicated and controversial. Poor quality mental health testimony can cause victimized children to go without protection and innocent defendants to be convicted. It is imperative that mental health testimony adhere to best practices.

Because accurate expert testimony is so critical, Kathryn Kuehnle and Mary Connell's 2009 book *The Evaluation of Child Sexual Abuse Allegations: A Comprehensive Guide to Assessment and Testimony* is an important contribution to the literature. Bringing together many of the world's leading experts, Kuehnle and Connell's book materially advances the field. Yet, like any scholarly endeavor, aspects of Kuehnle and Connell's book are subject to critique and disagreement. Indeed, some points in their book are, to my way of thinking, not only open to debate but are just plain wrong.

In the special issue of *The Journal of Child Sexual Abuse,* Kathleen Faller and Mark Everson orchestrate a series of important articles by leading experts, articles that explore the weaknesses in Kuehnle and Connell's book. These two publications—Kuehnle and Connell's book and Faller and Everson's special issue of the *Journal*—represent scholarship at its best: highly intelligent people who care deeply about the truth challenging and debating one another. The fact that authors in the journal are "fighting it out" with authors in book is not something to regret. It is an occasion to celebrate. Such debate is how progress is achieved. Bravo to both "sides"! this article adds to the discussion by registering disagreement with selected aspects of three chapters in *The Evaluation of Child Sexual Abuse Allegations*.

HERMAN'S FALSE DICHOTOMY AND RELATED FOIBLES

Steve Herman's chapter (2009) titled "Forensic Child Sexual Abuse Evaluations: Accuracy, Ethics, and Admissibility" contains a great deal of information that is worthwhile. I am a big fan of Steve's work, particularly his 2005 article in *Law and Human Behavior* (Herman, 2005). Unfortunately, in his chapter in *The Evaluation of Child Sexual Abuse Allegations*, Herman makes what I believe are five mistakes.

Herman's first mistake is the false dichotomy he draws between what he calls "hard" and "soft" evidence of sexual abuse. Herman writes, "Forensic evaluators base their judgments about the validity of allegations or suspicions of child sexual abuse (CSA) on two types of evidence: (1) hard evidence such as perpetrator confessions, medical evidence, photographs or videos of the abuse, and other physical evidence and (2) soft psychosocial evidence" (p. 247). Herman suggests "hard" evidence helps in the search for truth, but "soft" evidence does not. Where do the definitions of "hard" and "soft" come from? Herman cites no authority for his definitions.

Herman compounds the problem by making his second mistake—he equates the "soft psychosocial evidence" he deplores with children's verbal descriptions of abuse. What is "hard" about a perpetrator's confession and "soft" about a child's statement describing abuse? Is Herman suggesting perpetrator confessions are valid and children's statements are not? Surely that cannot be his intent. Some perpetrator confessions are true, and some are not. The same is so for children's statements. Herman does nothing to explain why a perpetrator confession is "hard" evidence worthy of credit while a child's description of abuse is "soft" evidence subject to doubt. Some perpetrator confessions are blatant lies intended to curry favor with authorities, and some statements by children provide compelling evidence of abuse.

To continue the critique of the false dichotomy between "hard" and "soft" evidence, why does medical evidence qualify as "hard"? Anyone familiar with the literature knows the controversy that has surrounded the interpretation of medical evidence. Medical evidence is neither "hard" nor "soft." In the final analysis, "hard" and "soft" are meaningless. Some medical evidence is powerful, some isn't.

Herman's third and fourth errors lie in his statement that "If there is clear and convincing hard evidence that either corroborates or contradicts an abuse allegation, then the soft psychosocial evidence is superfluous for the purpose of judging the validity of an abuse allegation" (p. 248). Herman states, "The term corroborated is used here in a narrower sense—consistent with law enforcement usage—to refer only to reports that are supported by hard evidence" (p. 248, footnote 1). Herman cites no authority for his assertion that "law enforcement usage" of corroborative evidence is limited to "hard evidence." I know of no such authority and believe Herman is simply wrong. In law, the term *corroborate* simply means strengthen. The Illinois Supreme Court defined corroboration in *In re A.P.* (1997): "To 'corroborate' means to add weight or credibility to a thing by additional and confirming facts or evidence, and 'corroborating evidence' means evidence supplementary to that already given and tending to strengthen or confirm it" (p. 650). Herman unintentionally misleads when he asserts that only "hard" evidence—whatever that is—is corroborative. Any evidence—"soft" or "hard"—that strengthens a proposition is corroborative.

To make matters worse, Herman asserts that if there is "hard" corroborative evidence—as he uses that term—then "soft psychosocial evidence is superfluous for the purpose of judging the validity of an abuse allegation." This statement is indefensible. Remember, Herman categorizes children's descriptions of abuse as "soft psychosocial evidence." Even when there is a plethora of "hard" evidence, a child's statements—and, I would argue, other psychosocial evidence—can provide evidence of abuse. To suggest that a child's statement describing abuse is "superfluous" when there is "hard" evidence is to suggest that such statements have no evidentiary value, a statement that finds no support in the literature, that seems illogical on its face, and that runs counter to centuries of law and experience relying on what witnesses say. Obviously, it can be difficult to evaluate the truthfulness of children's statements (and adults' statement too), and some statements are inaccurate, but to suggest that children's statements are "superfluous" is both wrong and dangerous.

Herman's fifth error is a large one. He asserts it is "faulty" to make inferences "about the validity of abuse allegations on the basis of psychosocial evidence, including children's reports in investigative interviews. The objection is not to investigative interviewing but to one use that is often made of data collected in investigative interviews: to make validity judgments. Investigative interviews are critical elements of good forensic CSA evaluations, but the purpose of such interviews should be to elicit information that is designed to lead to obtaining or discovering hard evidence that either supports or contradicts an abuse allegation" (Herman, 2009, p. 258). Is Herman suggesting children's interview statements have no probative value other than as clues to "hard" evidence, and only "hard" evidence counts? Of course, as already discussed, the dichotomy between "hard" and "soft" evidence is a false dichotomy, but to suggest that children's statements describing abuse have no probative value is absurd. Moreover, if Herman is right (he isn't), then he has another problem: How can he trust that children's statements—unreliable "psychosocial evidence"—will be valid clues to the "hard" evidence he wants so badly?

These errors are serious, and they are dangerous. The errors might be ignorable if they were made by a less influential commentator in a less important book, but they are not. Steve Herman is a well-intended, smart, leading authority on child sexual abuse. If I am right—even partly right—then Steve should correct his mistakes before his words hurt somebody.

AHERN, BRIDGES, AND FAUST—DOUBLE-DIPPING

The first three chapters of *The Evaluation of Child Sexual Abuse Allegations* are authored by David Ahern, Ana Bridges, and David Faust (Bridges, Faust, & Ahern, 2009; Faust, Bridges, & Ahern, 2009a, 2009b). The chapters are important contributions to the field; in particular, Ahern, Bridges, and Faust do a nice job explaining base rates.[3] One aspect of Chapters 2 and 3, however, "The Problem of Double-Dipping," appears to me to be either a miscommunication or a mistake that could lead to serious errors in practice.

Ahern, Bridges, and Faust explain double-dipping as follows: "Double-dipping occurs when an indicator [variable] is used . . . as a screening basis for referral for abuse evaluations, and is then used again during . . . evaluation. The problem is that once the variable or variables have been used during [the screening phase], then any positive qualities they might have had for the detection of abuse are neutralized when they are reapplied" during the evaluation (Bridges, Faust & Ahern, 2009, p. 29). The authors go on to say, "Once a valid and differentiating variable has already been used as a basis for referral, that variable losses its differentiating value because all children who are referred . . . demonstrate the characteristic. . . . [V]ariables used as a basis for referral lose their efficacy during the evaluation phase" (Faust, Bridges & Ahern, 2009b, p. 52).

Consider 6-year-old Sally. One day in her kindergarten class, Sally tries to insert a toy into her vagina. She tells her teacher, "Billy stuck his weiner in me. His weiner spit on me." Sally is referred for evaluation for possible sexual abuse. In the evaluation, is it proper for the evaluator to consider Sally's disclosure to the teacher and her act of attempting to insert a toy into her vagina? Do the child's statement and conduct have probative value for the evaluator? Bridges, Faust, and Ahern write, "Variables used as a basis for referral lose their efficacy during the evaluation phase." Do Bridges, Faust, and Ahern suggest the evaluator should ignore Sally's words and conduct? Do they mean Sally's words and conduct have lost their "differentiating value"?

I have read, re-read, and re-re-read Bridges, Faust, and Aherns' manuscripts, trying to understand their "double-dipping" argument. David Faust was kind enough to patiently walk me through the argument. For me, Sally's words and conduct are powerful evidence of sexual abuse at initial referral *and* at evaluation. Obviously, an evaluator should not count Sally's words and conduct twice, but to suggest that her words and conduct are somehow irrelevant at evaluation is preposterous. If Bridges, Faust, and Ahern really mean "variables used as a basis for referral lose their efficacy during the evaluation phase," then a diagnosing physician should not consider a patient's medical history. A police detective should disregard evidence discovered by the first police officer on the scene of the crime. Bridges, Faust, and Ahern cannot intend these results. If they do, then I respectfully submit they are wrong. The suggestion that evidence considered at referral is irrelevant at evaluation flies in the face of common sense and experience. On the other hand, if they are trying to say there is danger in overvaluing evidence used at initial screening, then I concur.

If I have misunderstood what Bridges, Faust, and Ahern's are saying—or are trying to say—then shame on me. I worry, however, that if I came away confused by their double-dipping argument, others might too. I worry frontline mental health professionals, social workers, lawyers, police officer, and judges might conclude from Bridges, Faust, and Ahern that they should disregard as evidence anything that constitutes "variables used as a basis for referral." This would be a dangerous mistake, because evidence used as a basis for referral remains relevant evidence. I conclude Bridges, Faust, and Ahern's double-dipping presentation iterates an error or is confusing. In either case, they should correct the problem so practitioners are not misled.

Mark Everson and Kathleen Faller (2012) critique the double-dipping argument in their article titled "Base Rates, Multiple Indicators, and Comprehensive Forensic Evaluations: Why Sexualized Behavior Still Counts in Assessments of Child Sexual Abuse Allegations." Thomas Lyon, Elizabeth Ahern, and Nicholas Scurich (2012) also address double-dipping in their article titled "Interviewing Children vs. Tossing Coins: Accurately Assessing the Diagnosticity of Children's Disclosure of Abuse."

I tip my hat to the editors of contributors to *The Evaluation of Child Sexual Abuse Allegations* and the *Journal of Child Sexual Abuse*. Thank you. You have moved us forward.

NOTES

1. To be admissible in court, evidence must be "relevant," that is the evidence must have some tendency in logic to prove a point that is raised in the case. All relevant evidence is admissible in court unless excluded by a particular rule or policy. For example, hearsay may be relevant but inadmissible under the rule against hearsay evidence.

2. Hearsay is a statement made prior to court proceedings (out of court) that is repeated in court to prove that the out of court statement is true. See Myers (2011).

3. Equally valuable insights into base rates are available in this issue of the *Journal of Child Sexual Abuse*. See Mark Everson and Kathleen Faller (2012) and Thomas Lyon, Elizabeth Ahern, and Nicholas Scurich (2012).

REFERENCES

Bridges, A. J., Faust, D., & Ahern D. C. (2009). Methods for the identification of sexually abused children: Reframing the clinician's task and recognizing its disparity with research on indicators (pp. 21–47). In K. Kuehnle & M. Connell (Eds.), *The evaluation of child sexual abuse allegations: A comprehensive guide to assessment and testimony*. New York: Wiley.

Everson, M. D., & Faller, K. C. (2012). Base rates, multiple indicators, and comprehensive forensic evaluations: Why sexualized behavior still counts in assessments of child sexual abuse allegations. *Journal of Child Sexual Abuse*, *21*(1), 45–71.

Faust, D., Bridges, A. J., & Ahern, D. C. (2009a). Methods for the identification of sexually abused children: Issues and needed features for abuse indicators. (pp. 3–19). In K. Kuehnle & M. Connell (Eds.), *The evaluation of child sexual abuse allegations: A comprehensive guide to assessment and testimony*. New York: Wiley.

Faust, D., Bridges, A. J., & Ahern, D. C. (2009b). Methods for the identification of sexually abused children: Suggestions for clinical work and research. (pp. 49–66). In K. Kuehnle & M. Connell (Eds.), *The evaluation of child sexual abuse allegations: A comprehensive guide to assessment and testimony*. New York: Wiley.

Herman, S. (2005). Improving decision making in forensic child sexual abuse evaluations. *Law and Human Behavior*, *29*(1), 87–120.

Herman, S. (2009). Forensic child sexual abuse evaluations: Accuracy, ethics, and admissibility. (pp. 247–266). In K. Kuehnle & M. Connell (Eds.), *The evaluation of child sexual abuse allegations: A comprehensive guide to assessment and testimony*. New York: Wiley.

In re A.P., 688 N.E.2d 642 (Ill. 1997).

In re Nicole V., 518 N.E.2d 914 (N.Y. 1987).

Kuehnle, K., & Connell, M. (Eds.). (2009). *The evaluation of child sexual abuse allegations: A comprehensive guide to assessment and testimony*. New York: Wiley.

Lyon, T. D., Ahern, E. C., & Scurich, N. (2012). Interviewing children vs. tossing coins: Accurately assessing the diagnosticity of children's disclosure of abuse. *Journal of Child Sexual Abuse, 21*(1), 19–44.

Melton, G. B. & Limber, S. (1989). Psychologists' involvement in cases of child maltreatment. *American Psychologist, 44*(9), 1225–1233.

Melton, G. B., Petrila, J., Poythress, N. G., & Slobogin, C. (2007). *Psychological evaluations for the courts: A handbook for mental health professionals and lawyers* (3rd ed.). New York: Guilford.

Myers, J. E. B. (2010). Expert testimony in child sexual abuse litigation: Consensus and confusion. *U.C. Davis Journal of Juvenile Law & Policy, 14*, 1–57.

Myers, J. E. B. (2012). *Myers on evidence of interpersonal violence: Child maltreatment, intimate partner violence, rape, stalking, and elder abuse*. New York: Aspen Law and Business.

Pennsylvania v. Ritchie, 480 U.S. 39 (1987).

AUTHOR NOTE

John E. B. Myers, JD, is a professor of law at the University of the Pacific, McGeorge School of Law in Sacramento, California.

Comment on Cross, Fine, Jones, and Walsh (2012): Do Mental Health Professionals Who Serve on/with Child Advocacy Centers Experience Role Conflict?

COLLEEN FRIEND
*California State University Los Angeles Child Abuse and Family Violence Institute,
Los Angeles, California, USA*

Cross, Fine, Jones, and Walsh's (2012) article "Mental Health Professionals in Children's Advocacy Centers: Is There Role Conflict?" challenges two recent publications' criticisms that child advocacy centers create role conflict for mental health professionals and explains how child advocacy centers actually work, describing the different roles for mental health professionals who participate in them. This commentary points out that more precise data would have helped to specifically address the critics' concerns. Furthermore, professional ethics and licensure issues may have served as an additional but unacknowledged check on the "spillover effect" that the critics have alleged comes with being associated with prosecution. This commentary also highlights three main strengths of the Cross and colleagues' article.

Child advocacy centers (CACs) provide comprehensive, multidisciplinary investigation and intervention for allegations of child sexual abuse (CSA) or other serious child abuse. Cross, Fine, Jones, and Walsh (2012) point out that coordinating the functions of criminal justice, mental health, child welfare, medical, victim advocacy, and other professionals is perhaps the most important function CACs serve. Cross and colleagues' article serves two functions: first, it argues that two recent publications' concerns that CACs create role conflict for mental health professionals overestimate the risk for this occurrence, and, second, it takes the position that a fundamental misunderstanding of CAC practices is a core issue here and explains how CACs actually work. Cross and colleagues' article is important because, once raised, these concerns should be addressed; otherwise, the credibility of CACs could suffer. How well the article addresses this is the subject of this commentary.

The two recent publications alleging role conflict for mental health professionals in CACs are both chapters in professional texts that have broader focus on assessing children. The most recent publication, Connell's (2008) chapter on CACs, raises the following issues: (a) the primary goal of CACs is to have more successful prosecutions, which conflicts with the mental health professional's need to be neutral and objective; (b) prosecuting, truth seeking, protecting, and treating are incompatible efforts; and (c) there are concerns about the extended forensic evaluation. Connell's chapter also resurrects some arguments advanced by Melton and Kimbrough-Melton (2006).

Melton and Kimbrough-Melton (2006) also offer a different, tactical criticism that centers on the following points: (a) mental health treatment providers and forensic evaluators often perform the same functions; that is, they may perform all the interventions on which child protective services, law enforcement, and prosecutors rely; (b) even when these functions are separated, mental health professionals participate in prosecutorial decision making, and this association (more so if it is through employment) may compromise the mental health professional's ability to be therapeutic with the instant or other families; and (c) even when physically separated, problems of a possible "spillover effect" persist from proximity and contact with investigative staff and thus give rise to the appearance of bias.

Cross and colleagues (2012) clearly describe the sources relied on to answer the concerns raised by these "critics." Among them are: (a) the National Children's Alliance's (NCA) membership and practice standards for CACs as well as the CAC director's manual on mental health services; (b) a multisite evaluation of CAC(s) performed by some of the authors; (c) interviews with key informants who were current or former directors; and (d) some of the authors' own experiences in being CAC directors or members of NCA state or national boards. This is a sound approach for answering the concerns about role conflict, because the reader needs to first know if Cross and colleagues have the depth of practice experience to meet this challenge and if they have access to policies and data that back up their contentions. While they clearly do, both Cross and colleagues and the critics miss a few important steps along the way.

The first issue the reader is left wondering about is whether Cross and colleagues (2012) and the critics agree on who is a mental health professional. Fortunately, Cross and colleagues introduce their version early on, stating this category includes clinical social workers, psychologists, psychiatrists, psychiatric nurses, and licensed mental health counselors. This coincides with the National Alliance on Mental Illness (NAMI, 2010) definition, yet NAMI importantly includes the need for licensure for each of these professions. In contrast, the reader is left to surmise what Connell (2008) and Melton and Kimbrough-Melton (2006) mean when referring to mental health professionals. The latter uses the terms *therapist, clinician*, and *expert evaluator* interchangeably to describe mental health professionals. To add to this confusion, when who is a mental health professional is reintroduced, Cross and colleagues rely on professional self-identification from unpublished training data. While this is welcomed, it is not completely clear. For example, 9.6% of professionals trained at the CAC in Huntsville self-identified as mental health professionals; others may have had a mental health education (e.g., a BSW or MSW) but identified themselves as a forensic interviewer or protective services worker (Lieth, 2010, as cited in Cross et al., 2012).

Beyond this, Cross and colleagues (2012) could have raised the argument that all mental health professionals, such as those listed by NAMI, have to adhere to their own professional code of ethics. A brief review of the codes of ethics of the American Psychological Association, the American Association for Marriage and Family Therapy, and the National Association of Social Workers shows convergence on these general areas: ensuring informed consent, honoring client's rights, not acting outside of the scope of practice, avoiding exploiting trust, avoiding or refraining from dual relationships, respecting client's autonomy to make decisions, and protecting confidentiality. If the mental health professional were licensed, there would be additional incentives to abide by these ethics as well as local and state laws. Raising this argument could participate in a strategy to confront the critics' assertion that mental health professionals participate in prosecutorial decisions and are vulnerable to a "spillover effect."

In addition to overlooking mental health professionals' own ethics, there is only a brief mention of prosecutorial ethics. This comes in the context of refuting that prosecution and truth seeking are incompatible. According a publication of the American Bar Association (Joy & McMunigal, 2005), prosecutors are expected to act differently from defense and civil attorneys; they are ministers of justice, not simply advocates. Prosecutors are required to make an informal adjudication of guilt, assess the credibility of the witness, and pursue the truth (Gershman, 2001). While case law provides examples of some prosecutors who did not comport with these ethics, it seems that it would be very hard to finesse this obligation before so many observers on a team at a CAC. This would have been a stronger argument than the one provided. Furthermore, Cross and colleagues explain why prosecutors and mental health therapists would want and need to keep their distance from one another.

When Cross and colleagues (2012) were describing the mental health professionals' functions in relationship to a CAC, the authors used vague terms (e.g., "most," "often," "some," "typically," etc.) at least a dozen times when more specific data would have presumably shown the strength of their position. For example, the authors state that, "in the *overwhelming majority* of CACs, forensic interviewers never provide treatment to CAC clients, and therapists working with CAC clients never conduct forensic interviews" (p. 97, emphasis added). What does "overwhelming majority" mean? As if to explain, the authors then offer, "In a *very small number* of CACs, mental health professionals conduct forensic interviews on some cases and provide treatment on others, but even then, the same professional does not perform both functions with the same child" (p. 97, emphasis added). What is that "very small number"? Why is this information so obscure if they just completed a multisite study? Along these same lines, in an effort to assert that CACs are not as prosecution-oriented as the critics suggest, the reader gets more imprecise language, "*most* CACs are independent non-profit organizations, and *many* are hospital-based or part of larger non-profits" (p. 102, emphasis added). Why not let the reader see the exact percentages on this from the author's data? Although Cross and colleagues (2012) provide some clarity on the variety of roles a mental health professional might serve in, they also contradict themselves by proclaiming, "Therapists *are not involved* in the initial investigation team" (p. 98, emphasis added). A few pages later, the reader is told that "children's therapists *rarely, if ever participate* in the investigation team" (p. 101, emphasis added).

Despite the confusion about who is a mental health professional, the nonspecificity about professional ethical standards, and the use of imprecise terms, Cross and colleagues (2012) present an important general picture of how CACs operate, especially in the ways that mental health professionals are utilized. They then outline several rebuttals or counterclaims to the critics' assertions. Strongest among them is the separation of the forensic interviewer and therapist function for the same child, followed by evidence that prosecution is not the primary purpose of a CAC, and wrapping up with explaining how a therapist's support for a family that is aligned with prosecution is good practice. First, the insistence on separating the interviewer and therapist roles did not emerge with CACs; recommendations for separation have existed since at least the second edition of the *Psychosocial Evaluation of Suspected Abuse in Children* guidelines by the American Professional Association on the Abuse of Children (APSAC, 1997). The authors refer to the NCA standards requiring this, and the reference list shows a 2008 publication date for revised standards, but the previous edition's standard insisted on this as well. The history of this tradition is not provided and would have made the authors' case stronger. Next, the authors eloquently describe why prosecution is not the primary goal of the CAC movement. CACs reflect national prosecution rates, which have hovered at about 10% for child abuse over the past decade (Cross, Walsh, Simone, & Jones, 2003). Cross and colleagues (2012) persuasively show how the CAC model considers both prosecution and therapeutic outcomes, not either/or. The authors are correct in noting that CACs deliver more in the capacity of child protection, advocacy, and mental health treatment services. Finally, the authors mount a persuasive argument that good mental health practice calls for engaging and supporting the child and family through the path they would be choosing to take and that avoidance of all or some contact with other system professionals, such as prosecutors, perhaps in the service of not having any appearance of role conflict, would do their clients a disservice.

The critics would not have had access to either the multisite evaluation (Cross et al., 2008) or the joint report issued by the National Child Traumatic Stress Network and NCA (2008). If they had, would their conclusions be different? The latter publication is careful to report on what forensic interviewers (who may also be trained mental health professionals) do with the caregiver/parent: they share their professional opinion regarding the risk to the child and report any alleged offenders the child identified. Then they help the caregiver/parent manage that feedback so he or she can help the child cope (National Child Traumatic Stress Network & National Children's Alliance, 2008). Once that initial investigation is complete, law enforcement and child protective services may decrease their contact, and this may be the time that the family begins to transition from the forensic team to the mental health professional. The mental health professional is likely to form a strong, consistent, and trusting relationship with the parent as well as the child. The literature clearly shows that the nonoffending caregiver/parent's response to the child in the wake of CSA (or other serious abuse) is critical to the psychosocial adjustment of the child victim (Conte & Schuerman, 1987; Deblinger, Steer, & Lippman, 1999). The irony here is that parental support of the child is ultimately what the child perceives and remembers the most, long after professionals banter about role confusion.

Cross and colleagues (2012) did not address Connell's (2008) concerns about the extended forensic evaluation. Although this might not be specifically related to mental health role conflict, this pioneering CAC initiated approach aimed to reach about one-fourth of the children interviewed at CACs (Faller & Nelson-Gardell, 2010) with a structured, multisession protocol that deserves defending as one of the many ways CACs have moved all of our professions ahead in the service of the child's needs over the convenience of the system.

In the end, Cross and colleagues (2012) and the critics agree in calling for more research about how professionals actually function within a multidisciplinary team. Cross and colleagues then describe the beginnings of a multiple method protocol for doing just that. This would be a welcome contribution to the field; we hope the Office of Juvenile Justice and Delinquency Prevention, funders of the multisite evaluation of CACs, are listening.

REFERENCES

American Professional Association on the Abuse of Children. (1997). *Psychosocial evaluation of suspected abuse in children* (2nd ed.). Chicago: Author.

Connell, M. (2008). The child advocacy center model. In K. Kuehnle & M. Connell (Eds.), *The evaluation of child sexual abuse allegations: A comprehensive guide to assessment and testimony* (pp. 423–429). New York: Wiley.

Conte, J. & Schuerman, J. (1987). The effects of sexual abuse on children: A multidimensional view. *Journal of Interpersonal Violence, 2,* 380–390.

Cross, T. P., Fine, J. E., Jones, L. M., and Walsh, W. A. (2012). Mental health professionals in children's advocacy centers: Is there role conflict? *Journal of Child Sexual Abuse, 21*(1), 91–108.

Cross, T. P., Jones, L. J., Walsh, W., Simone, M., Kolko, D. J., Szczepanski, J., et al. (2008). *The multi-site evaluation of children's advocacy centers: Executive summary: Findings from the UNH multi-site evaluation of children's advocacy centers.* Bulletin. Washington DC: OJJDP Crimes Against Children Series.

Cross, T. P., Walsh, W., Simone, M., & Jones, L. M. (2003). Prosecution of child abuse: A meta- analysis of rates of criminal justice decisions. *Trauma, Violence and Abuse, 4,* 323–340.

Deblinger, E., Steer, R., & Lippman, J. (1999). Two year follow up study of cognitive behavioral therapy for sexually abused children suffering post-traumatic stress symptoms. *Child Abuse & Neglect, 23*(12), 1371–1378.

Faller, K., & Nelson- Gardell, D. (2010). Extended evaluations in cases of child sexual abuse: How many cases are sufficient? *Journal of Child Sexual Abuse, 19,* 648–668.

Gershman, B.L. (2001). The prosecutor's duty to truth. *Pace Law Faculty Publications, Paper 128.* Retrieved December 26, 2010, from http://digitalcommons.pace.edu/lawfaculty/128

Joy, P., & McMunigal, K. (2005). Why should prosecutors seek justice? *Criminal Justice Magazine, 20*(2). Retrieved December 22, 2012, from http://www.americanbar.org/publications/criminal_justice_magazine_home/crimjust_cjmag_20_2_home.html

Melton, G., & Kimbrough-Melton, R. (2006). Integrating assessment, treatment and justice: Pipe dream or possibility? In S. Sparta & G. Koocher (Eds.), *Forensic mental health assessments of children and adolescents* (pp. 30–45). New York: Oxford University Press.

National Alliance on Mental Illness. (2010). *Mental health professionals: Who they are and how to find one.* Retrieved December 26, 2010, from http://www.nami.org/Template.cfm?Section=Helpline&template=/ContentManagement/ContentDisplay.cfm&ContentID=4867

National Child Traumatic Stress Network & National Children's Alliance. (2008). *CAC director's guide to mental health services for abused children*. Los Angeles: National Center for Child Traumatic Stress.

AUTHOR NOTE

Colleen Friend, PhD, LCSW, is the director of the CSULA Child Sexual Abuse and Family Violence Institute in Los Angeles, California. She was the past director of both the Los Angeles County Child Abuse Crisis Center and Stuart House.

Comment on Cross, Fine, Jones, and Walsh (2012): We Are Now on the Same Page

SETH L. GOLDSTEIN
Private Practice, Monterey, California, USA

Role conflict has been an issue in the intervention of child abuse cases since the beginning of the alliance drawn between the legal and mental health professions. In child abuse cases, clearly defined roles will prevent an attack on the process, thereby providing successful interventions to protect children. The child advocacy center concept is one of the best ways to meld the two professional functions into a cohesive approach to those interventions.

In the third decade of the conceptual existence of a multidisciplinary team and ultimately the child advocacy center we are again talking about role conflicts. In the beginning, there was much concern about whether law enforcement and prosecutorial offices could successfully turn over the role of interviewing children to people who were not law enforcement personnel. There was no "team" concept, and services to abused children were adding to the trauma because of an often disjointed and repetitive process.

Before the idea of the multidisciplinary concept came to fruition, different agency objectives and roles caused conflicts and lack of trust between social workers and those in law enforcement. The role conflicts caused problems in the development of evidence and cases ultimately resulting in children not getting the services that were necessary or the protection that was required. Then came the day care and nursery school cases where law enforcement could not possibly handle the volume of interviews that were necessary, and they turned to members of the mental health community to assist in the assessment of information and, more important, securing statements from children who had been abused. The fallout from the well-intentioned efforts of all concerned set those relationships on edge, causing setbacks to the intervention of child sexual abuse cases.

What we have learned (and what was really the main issue in the beginning) is that role conflict is a constant and ever-present issue in the intervention in child abuse in general and in sexual abuse more particularly. It is necessary for each and every individual who assists in the development of evidence toward a prosecutorial goal to understand their role. They must know the limits of that role as well as the rules of the road they must follow.

In almost every case in which the involvement of a mental health professional has been called into question in the intervention of child abuse through a child advocacy center, the attack has been on qualifications, process, and a question about boundaries as it relates to the fact gatherer's role in the system. Both Melton and Kimbrough-Melton (2006) and Cross, Fine, Jones, and Walsh (2012) have it right: there must be clear boundaries and definitions of roles for those mental health professionals participating in the child advocacy center.

The child advocacy center is, and always has been, a means to obtain information in a legally defensible manner all the while supporting the child through the process. If done properly it reduces the number of interviews and provides a resource to follow the child through the ordeal. The successes of the multidisciplinary concept, be it in a formal child advocacy center setting or otherwise, tells us that we must constantly be aware of the errors of the past so as not to make the same mistakes again and lose the confidence that we developed in a system that works on behalf of children.

It cannot be emphasized enough: role definition is a critical element in the operation of a child advocacy center. The interviewers, be they mental health professionals or law enforcement, must know the rules of the road and stick to them. A therapist or other mental health professional cannot both counsel a child, the child's family, or anyone else in the case and also act as an independent, nonbiased seeker of truth. The therapeutic ethical codes of every level of mental health profession discourage multiple relationships (dual roles) because of the often conflicting expectations and pressures brought about by those roles.

Unfortunately, some therapeutic techniques have been called into question when they are used to elicit information from child victims. When securing information for a criminal or juvenile dependency (child protection) matter, the process must conform to reliable standards.

The reason why mental health professionals are often better suited to conduct interviews with children is because of their understanding of child development and the psychological impact of physical, psychological, and sexual trauma. They are also aware of the various psychological symptoms not just of trauma but also other maladies. During the interview process, they may be able to bring out evidence that would bear on the credibility of the statements made by a child who suffers from something other than or in combination with abuse.

The child advocacy center's information gathering function must be separate from therapy because therapists establish a relationship with their patient. Otherwise a therapist may be attacked on the basis of an inherent bias. This is another reason why there must be a separation between those who provide aid to the child and those who gather information. Therapists often become advocates for the children they see. The interview process is supposed to be a neutral setting where the object is to obtain the truth. There must be no relationship between the child and interviewer other than a professional meeting (or meetings[1]) to obtain information. If that neutrality is compromised, so too may be the information that comes from it.

Now, with the standards set by the National Child Advocacy Center, whether it be a law enforcement officer or a mental health professional, the interviewer has a clear view of what role he or she to play in the process. The therapeutic role is different from that of information gathering. A mental health professional working in a child advocacy center must not engage the child or the child's family in any relationship other than that of the professional fact gatherer associated with the child advocacy center. With this boundary made clear, both the mental health professional and the children they serve will benefit.

NOTE

1. The extended interview is getting more press and must be seriously considered in cases of abuse in which children are reluctant to talk about what happened to them.

REFERENCES

Cross, T. P., Fine, J. E., Jones, L. M., and Walsh, W. A. (2012). Mental health professionals in children's advocacy centers: Is there role conflict? *Journal of Child Sexual Abuse*, *21*(1), 91–108.

Melton, G. B., & Kimbrough-Melton, R. J. (2006). Integrating assessment, treatment, and justice: Pipe dream or possibility. In S. N. Sparta & G. P. Koocher (Eds.), *Forensic mental health assessment of children and adolescents* (pp. 30–45). New York: Oxford University Press.

AUTHOR NOTE

Seth L. Goldstein, Esq., is a California attorney in private practice handling child abuse cases in the civil, family law and juvenile courts. He also represents mental health professionals in licensing and discipline matters. He was also a law enforcement officer, serving as a co-chairman of an early multidisciplinary team. He is the author of *The Sexual Exploitation of Children: A Practical Guide to Assessment, Investigation and Intervention* (2nd ed., CRC Press, 1999).

Comment on Cross, Fine, Jones, and Walsh (2012): Good Therapeutic Services—Therapeutic Advocacy and Forensic Neutrality

MARY CONNELL
Independent Practice, Fort Worth, Texas, USA

Cross, Fine, Jones, and Walsh (2012) provided a thoughtful review and critique of a book chapter describing the interview process at Child Advocacy Centers. They observed some of the ways that concerns raised in that chapter are being addressed and described revised guidelines that further clarify issues. Ongoing research and examination of the important processes carried on by child advocacy centers and the role fulfilled by mental health professionals in the investigation of child sexual abuse contributes positively to service delivery.

In their timely and thought-provoking article, Cross, Fine, Jones, and Walsh (2012) offer an updated perspective on potential role conflicts for mental health professionals who serve Child Advocacy Centers (CACs). This is a critically important issue for anyone seeking to proffer or review evidence in cases involving allegations of child abuse.

In prior book chapters addressing a range of CAC-related clinical and forensic issues, Melton and Kimbrough-Melton (2006) and Connell (2009a) commented on existing role conflict standards and related concerns. Since that time, the National Advocacy Center has adopted the National Children's Alliance (NCA) Standards for Accredited Members Revised 2011. These standards now clarify the role boundaries of mental health professionals at

CACs (National Children's Alliance, 2011) and set forth clear role definitions and mechanisms for ensuring independence, autonomy, and coordination of services among the participants of the multidisciplinary team.

STRENGTHENING AND CLARIFYING THE DISTINCTION BETWEEN INVESTIGATION AND TREATMENT

Cross and colleagues (2012) describe how mental health services are separated from the investigative process in the actual functioning of most CACs. They correctly identify some of the issues raised by Melton and Kimbrough-Melton (2006) and Connell (2009a) as moot. For example, they note that CAC forensic interviewers may or may not be mental health service providers but when conducting forensic interviews are serving an investigative rather than mental health function. Some mental health providers also serve as consultants but do not provide investigative or treatment services. Mental health providers who are providing therapy may not serve at all on the investigative multidisciplinary team (MDT) and may have fairly limited involvement in team decisions as the case advances. Therapeutic and investigative efforts are distinct, and when therapists provide input it is often to voice the concerns or preferences of the child or family or to assist in determining how best to protect the child's well-being during testimony. However, some concerns remain about roles, which will be described here after a brief look at how the revised standards address the boundaries of mental health professionals at CACs.

Some points clarifying the role of the mental health professional in CACs that were explicated in the revised standards (National Children's Alliance, 2008) bear particular mention:

1. The revised standards (p. 8) distinguish between the role of the forensic interviewer and the role of the therapist. NCA standards state that "every effort should be made to maintain clear boundaries between these roles and processes" (p. 26). The standards require each CAC to document in writing how the forensic process is separate from mental health treatment. This direct and clear division of the two services was not explicitly addressed in the prior standards. The closest parallel in the 2003 standards was found under Therapeutic Services—Rated Criteria (G): "The forensic interview or assessment is separate from mental health treatment" (p. 11).
2. Mental health treatment is defined in the revised standards as a clinical process designed to assess and mitigate the long-term adverse impact of trauma or other diagnosable mental health conditions. This definition was not offered in the 2003 standards, which instead listed among the components necessary for membership in the NCA: "Therapeutic Intervention: Specialized mental health services are to be made available as part of the

team response, either at the CAC or through coordination and referral with other appropriate treatment providers" (p. 2), without explicating the purpose of the mental health services. The clarification of purpose and inclusion of the definition of mental health treatment in the revised standards is a positive advancement.
3. In the revised standards is the following language clarifying the focus of mental health treatment services:

> Without effective therapeutic intervention, many traumatized children will suffer ongoing or long-term adverse social, emotional, and developmental outcomes that may impact them throughout their lifetimes. Today we have evidenced-based treatments and other practices with strong empirical support that will both reduce the impacts of trauma and the risk of future abuse. For these reasons, an MDT response must include trauma assessment and specialized trauma-focused mental health services for child victims and non-offending family members. (p. 22)

This focus on the unique therapeutic needs of traumatized children and emphasis on evidence-based treatment and other practices with strong empirical support reflects awareness of the importance of using research to advance the services offered through CACs.
4. Provisions are made in the standards regarding how the mental health treatment provider can share relevant information with the MDT while protecting the client's right to confidentiality and protecting the mental health records, to the extent possible. The revised standards make specific mention of the client's right to confidentiality (to the extent possible) and professional ethics in the context of information sharing—the 2003 standards included a generic statement regarding sharing of confidential information but did not specifically address confidentiality of mental health records. The standards explicate that CACs are expected to maintain at least minimal data on the mental health referral, including status and outcome, to be included in twice annual updates of statistical information to the NCA. The standards do not call for extensive data sharing.

SEPARATING INVESTIGATION FROM INTERVENTION

These clear efforts to separate the investigative process from the treatment process are excellent; however, in actual practice the boundaries may be difficult to maintain. An example may illustrate the problem. The mental health treatment provider presumably wishes to retain neutrality on the question of whether an alleged abuse incident actually occurred when it is disputed and provides supportive and helpful treatment during the pendency of the investigation and legal management of the case (Kuehnle & Connell, 2011). The standards anticipate, however, that as participants in the mainstay case review process, mental health treatment providers will, among other duties, provide input for prosecution and sentencing decisions (National Children's Allliance, p. 27). The mental health provider who shares observations and articulates the child's or family's concerns or wishes may be operating absolutely consistently with the therapist's role; the mental health provider who takes on the task of cultivating further investigative information in therapy sessions is not operating within a separate and clearly defined therapeutic role.

THE THERAPIST ASSISTING PROSECUTION OR CHILD PROTECTION EFFORTS

In examining how therapists might interact with prosecution and child protection efforts, the authors state:

> If therapists have assessed children's and caregivers' wishes and their interests accurately, and secured children's assent and non-offending caregivers' informed consent, there are circumstances in which it is appropriate for therapists to join with the family to assist prosecution and child protection professionals. It would be a misleading overstatement to describe this as being "actively engaged as prosecutorial investigators" since it mostly involves either appropriately sharing information or supporting children and families in the legal process.
>
> With the child and family's consent and support, therapists may be able to share information from the treatment that would assist investigation or prosecution, such as observations of child behavior that might reflect the impact of abuse. Therapists may also be able to assist both children and prosecutors appropriately if cases go to trial. For example, therapists may advise prosecutors about when children may be emotionally ready to testify and may suggest strategies to help prepare a child for the courtroom experience. They may serve as an extra support person in court for the child and, at sentencing, may work with victim witness advocates and the child to prepare a developmentally appropriate victim impact statement. (pp. 101–102)

And later the authors note:

> The CAC investigation method assumes that *the accuracy of the allegation is unknown* at the outset. This is a principle that is critical to criminal prosecution given the high standard of proof and the ensuing potential

consequences (i.e., loss of liberty) for those accused. Truth-seeking serves the goal of successful prosecution and is not undermined by it. (p. 102, italics added for emphasis)

Kuehnle and Connell (2011) have argued that the therapist should maintain the assumption that "the accuracy of the allegation is unknown" until the fact-finder makes a determination. To the extent that the child sees the therapist assisting prosecutors, advocating regarding the child's preparedness to testify, and supporting the child in court, the child may assume the therapist is joining the team in an effort to prosecute the alleged perpetrator. This may cause problems in the therapeutic alliance between child and therapist if the child still is attached and loves the perpetrator or if it is a case of a false positive and the child is not a victim of sexual abuse.

A CONSENSUS ON ROLE CONFLICT

Cross and colleagues (2012) particularly excell in describing the functioning of CACs and the roles of mental health professionals in them. In light of their observations and the revised standards, it appears that most of the concerns about potential role conflict have been addressed. However, as Cross and colleagues note, there is a dearth of research on how mental health professionals actually do function in CACs, which, as the authors note, is indeed an empirical question; studies are needed in this area. The authors observe that surveys of CACs could be conducted to produce descriptive statistics on how mental health professionals participate in MDTs and other CAC functions and specifically how CACs guard the boundaries between the roles of forensic interviewer and therapist. Cross and colleagues suggest two or three methods that could explore how mental health professionals function in CACs, in what ways they communicate and collaborate with other disciplines, and how they interact in team meetings. They suggest that it might be useful to solicit and study examples of cases or events in which role conflict occurred or there was a risk of role conflict and study the resulting sample of case examples. As the authors aptly note, boundary confusion can happen within or apart from the CAC structure, and the interests of both the child and of justice will be well served by a sophisticated approach within CACs to identify and address this problem when it arises.

THE MENTAL HEALTH PROFESSIONAL AND THE EXTENDED FORENSIC EVALUATION

When a child who is suspected of being sexually abused does not make an allegation or provide sufficient detail for investigation of suspected sexual abuse, the child may be referred for an Extended Forensic Evaluation (EFE). The EFE is a series of interview sessions with the child for the purpose of providing the child an additional opportunity to disclose abuse in a safe place. The sessions of the EFE may be conducted at the CAC or through a privately contracted mental health provider or other interviewer and are much more likely to be confused, at least by the outside observer, as therapy. These sessions, in contrast to the forensic interview, are not typically audio or video recorded, and the number of sessions with the interviewer (usually 5–8) is sufficient to anticipate that a quasi-therapeutic relationship may emerge. Connell (2009b) explored some factors about the EFE that raise concerns and to the extent that mental health providers may conduct the EFE, concerns with role boundaries follow (those that dealt with other aspects of the EFE are beyond the scope of this commentary).

The EFE evaluator's role as a member of the MDT may be contrary to the independence or autonomy needed for an objective evaluation. To the extent that some, if not most, EFEs are conducted by mental health professionals, the methods often utilized in forensic assessment may be relevant (e.g., see American Psychological Association, 2011; Greenberg & Shuman, 1997; Heilbrun, 2001). These methods include maintenance of a position of objectivity or avoidance of bias, keeping records that may withstand judicial scrutiny or that transparently track what occurred during the evaluation, and retaining neutrality from trial advocacy.

Although this procedure is called an EFE, it differs in some substantial ways from a traditional forensic evaluation and the distinctions raise questions about the role of the EFE. There is no report prepared to document the evaluator's (or MDT's) review of data to determine that referral to an EFE is warranted; such a report might describe the formal forensic interview and other data, including the child's initial denials or equivocation and explicating the reason abuse is suspected or the alternative hypotheses under consideration. At the conclusion of the EFE, the evaluator apparently does not prepare a *typical* forensic report of evaluation. Such a report would traditionally include the basis for referral or referral questions; the documents reviewed by the evaluator, a full description of the data collected through interviews, collateral contacts, and other data collection procedures; a discussion of the data supporting or negating each of several hypotheses; and, if appropriate, findings or recommendations (whether supportive of the abuse hypothesis or not) along with a clear explication of the nexus between the data and the recommendations. Instead, the EFE evaluator prepares a final report detailing the evaluation and other investigatory data, but it is not clear whether this report becomes accessible for review during the judicial process. If not, it may be that different disciplines are using the term "forensic evaluation" very differently. The EFE may be an extension of the investigation, again raising concerns about role confusion if the EFE evaluator is a mental health professional.

There is no mention in the EFE model or training materials of audio or video recording EFE sessions. Furthermore, no research has been done to examine the EFE interview process for adherence to the EFE model or to best practices. It is essential that these sessions be audio-recorded in order to provide transparency in how the allegations arise and opportunities to research the efficacy of this extended forensic interviewing process.

GOALS SERVED BY COLLEGIAL REVIEW

Cross and colleagues (2012) adopt a thorough and thoughtful approach to the collection of data in order to review and respond to the concerns raised by Melton and Kimbrough-Melton (2006) and Connell (2009a). Ultimately, all of the authors are undoubtedly working toward the same goals: to ensure the integrity of the process by which these important investigations of possible child sexual abuse are conducted and the constructive involvement in CACs by mental health professionals in the separate and distinct roles of forensic interviewer or therapist. We must all be concerned about how to intervene without compromising the evidence. In no other crime, perhaps, is the victim's statement so pivotal to the ultimate legal resolution. It may be devastating for children who have been abused and their families to endure a lengthy legal case only to witness an acquittal because of problems in the collection and preservation of evidence or for the child inaccurately identified as sexually abused to lose the relationship of an innocent parent or loved one. The child's account is often the single most important piece of evidence and it is critically important that everyone who speaks with a child about alleged abuse be mindful of the risk of altering the child's account or memory and thwarting a just legal outcome. As there is little organized feedback from the legal system to the frontline investigators and others who become involved with the case, well-intentioned but disastrous errors may continue unabated. When we can talk about and engage in research on ways to improve the process, the best interests of the child and the goals of justice can be achieved.

REFERENCES

American Psychological Association. (2001). *Specialty guidelines for forensic psychology*. Retrieved from http://www.apa.org/practice/guidelines/forensic-psychology.aspx

Connell, M. (2009a). The child advocacy center model. In K. Kuehnle & M. Connell (Eds.), *The evaluation of child sexual abuse allegations: A comprehensive guide to assessment and testimony* (pp. 423–449). New York: Wiley.

Connell, M. (2009b). The extended forensic evaluation. In K. Kuehnle & M. Connell (Eds.), *The evaluation of child sexual abuse allegations: A comprehensive guide to assessment and testimony* (pp. 451–487). New York: Wiley.

Cross, T. P., Fine, J. E., Jones, L. M., & Walsh, W. A. (2012). Mental health professionals in children's advocacy centers: Is there role conflict? *Journal of Child Sexual Abuse, 21*(1), 91–108.

Cross, T. P., Jones, L. J., Walsh, W., Simone, M., Kolko, D. J., Szczepanski, J., et al. (2008). *The multi-site evaluation of children's advocacy centers: Overview of the results and implications for practice.* Washington DC: OJJDP Crimes Against Children Series. Bulletin.

Greenberg, S., & Shuman, D. W. (1997). Irreconcilable conflict between therapeutic and forensic roles. *Professional Psychology: Research and Practice, 28*, 50–57.

Heilbrun, K. (2001). *Principles of forensic mental health assessment.* New York: Kluwer Academic/Plenum Press.

Kuehnle, K., & Connell, M. (2011). Managing children's emotional and clinical needs. In M. Lamb, D. La Rooy, C. Katz, &L. Malloy (Eds.), *Children's testimony: A handbook of pschological research and forensic practice* (2nd ed., pp. 179–199). London: Wiley-Blackwell.

Melton, G. B., & Kimbrough-Melton, R. J. (2006). Integrating assessment, treatment, and justice: Pipe dream or possibility. In S. N. Sparta & G. P. Koocher (Eds.), *Forensic mental health assessment of children and adolescents* (pp. 30–45). New York: Oxford University Press.

National Children's Alliance. (2011). *Standards for accredited members revised 2011.* Washington, DC: Author.

AUTHOR NOTE

Mary Connell, EdD, Independent Practice, Fort Worth, Texas.

A Response to Commentary on Faust, Bridges, and Ahern's (2009) "Methods for the Identification of Sexually Abused Children"

DAVID C. AHERN
Brown University, Providence, Rhode Island, USA

ANA J. BRIDGES
University of Arkansas, Fayetteville, Arkansas, USA

DAVID FAUST
University of Rhode Island, Kingston, Rhode Island, USA; and Brown University, Providence, Rhode Island, USA

Our series of three chapters (Faust, Bridges, & Ahern, 2009a, 2009b; Bridges, Faust, & Ahern, 2009) on the methodology of identifying sexually abused children elicited a number of comments, both supportive and critical. The criticisms appear related to three primary issues or apparent misconceptions of our work, perhaps due in part to incomplete exposition or ambiguity in presented material: our use of hypotheticals, our argument against "double-dipping," and our use of Bayesian analyses. We address each of these criticisms here in the hope of clarifying any misunderstandings and contributing in a constructive way to progress in this critical arena.

We appreciate this opportunity for an open exchange of ideas on a topic of utmost importance and to further the constructive ends all participants surely wish to achieve: to protect children while minimizing error and, thereby, harm. There is little doubt we are all striving to reach such ends, and we share in the fervent desire to enhance welfare.

For those unfamiliar with our three chapters (Faust, Bridges, & Ahern, 2009a, 2009b; Bridges, Faust, & Ahern, 2009), we wish to start by providing some context that may help in framing issues. Our chapters describe a wide range of principles and procedures for performing assessment and enhancing the accuracy of clinical decision making. Potential limits and problems in a range of methods are discussed, but solely for constructive reasons. To the extent clinicians and researchers understand the strengths and limits of measurement tools and decision strategies, weaker methods may be replaced with better methods and research efforts may be directed toward overcoming limits, enhancing strengths, and circumventing obstacles to more accurate assessment. Our chapters are certainly not limited to criticisms but also set forth numerous principles and strategies to enhance decision making, and we devote considerable attention to research approaches we believe hold promise for increasing knowledge and the efficacy of assessment methods. Understandably, it might not be apparent that other authors took issue with only a small minority of the points we raise, which suggests there may be considerably greater common ground than might otherwise seem to be the case.

In this commentary, we address what we view to be the main criticisms, which seem to stem largely from three misconceptions relating to (a) our use of hypotheticals, (b) the "double-dipping" problem, and (c) our Bayesian analyses. Each is explored in turn in this article. To the extent our arguments were potentially misunderstood, we recognize the fault may lie in our lucidity of expression or insufficient explication, and we welcome this chance to clarify certain matters.

HYPOTHETICALS AS LITERAL

In our chapters, we frequently use hypothetical examples to illustrate key principles. Unfortunately, it appears there was a tendency to take these hypotheticals literally or as factual assertions, perhaps because we did not sufficiently and explicitly stress the theoretical or supposed nature of our illustrations, something we took as evident. There are, of course, various potential uses of hypothetical assumptions. In areas such as child abuse, one often uses hypotheticals because certain facts are not well known or are in dispute and yet the principles of interest nevertheless hold across a wide range of possibilities, almost regardless of what the specifics may be. For example, if one wants to illustrate the negative impact of a weak or invalid variable on decision making, the importance of the argument or principle does not change regardless of the hypothetical variable used for expository purposes. Similarly, whether different values, proportions, or vocabulary are substituted—say, "nail biting" or "hair twirling" in place of "overt sexual behaviors"—the underlying principles of our arguments remain unchanged.

Our emphasis is on the validity, differentiating value, and augmenting value of any particular indicator, whatever the indicator happens to be.

Of course, if a reader mistakes hypotheticals as factual assertions, it is natural to raise criticisms or concerns when these presumed facts seem mistaken. We often employ examples within the domain of child sexual abuse because of the content we address. We generally tried to remain within the broad bounds of realistic possibilities, but the extent to which we may or may not have achieved this aim does not bear on the merits or applications of the principles of decision making we describe.

The distinction between the use of hypotheticals for illustrative purposes and factual assertions is of particular concern because of the perceived notion we dismiss any potential value of specific indicators out of hand. For example, Everson and Faller (2012) contend we condemn "the field of forensic assessment for its 'unwarranted' use of sexualized behavior and other behavioral symptoms as possible indicators or evidence of sexual abuse" (p. 46). Furthermore, in reference to our chapters, Everson and Faller argue, "the authors cite the 'unverified' and 'limited' diagnostic value of such behavior indicators and the 'grave' risk of false-positive decision errors inherent in their use" (p. 46). However, our intent is to explicate that any variable or predictor, regardless of its nature, is inappropriate to use when lacking any or all of the criteria we set forth. If an indicator lacks validity, lacks differentiating value, or lacks augmenting value, then the indicator is a poor or "unwarranted" choice. However, if a variable or indictor possesses all three characteristics, then inclusion in diagnostic decision making is justified whether such an indicator is behavioral, cognitive, or otherwise defined.

Our hypothetical examples focus almost exclusively on behavioral indicators, perhaps giving rise to this confusion. However, as we stated in Chapter 1, "Methods for the Identification of Sexually Abused Children" (Faust, Bridges, & Ahern, 2009a):

> The first necessary characteristic of an indicator variable for child sexual abuse is validity. In this context, valid means an association between that variable and the occurrence of child sexual abuse. In the context of mental health evaluations, our focus is typically on the possible association between abuse and some type of behavioral, affective, or cognitive outcome. *If* child sexual abuse produces or increases hypervigilance, then there is a true or valid association between sexual abuse and hypervigilance. Of course, other variables mental health professionals might justifiably consider to be within their purview, such as an increase in certain somatic complaints, may be validly associated with child sexual abuse. *Nevertheless, for now we will focus on behavioral, affective, and cognitive consequences, because limiting the analysis to such variables does not alter any of the principles or points that follow.* (p. 6, emphasis added)

We do not wish to criticize or condemn the use of sexualized behavior or other behavioral symptoms in abuse evaluations *per se*. Rather, we support the use of variables that improve diagnostic or predictive accuracy. Although behavioral symptoms are the focus of our hypotheticals, the validity, differentiating value, and augmenting nature of an indicator are of utmost concern.

"DOUBLE-DIPPING"

We were distressed to learn that core elements of our assertions about "double-dipping" were almost completely misunderstood, and we take such communication gaps very seriously. What writer wishes a potentially helpful idea to come across to a reader as badly flawed, thereby potentially negating the idea's utility to achieve pro-social aims? Myers (this issue) contends our line of reasoning "iterates an error or is confusing," while Everson and Faller (2012) levy much stronger criticisms. The latter authors provide two examples to illustrate perceived errors in our argument. The first involves a hospital admission for chest pain:

> 1st year resident to ER patient, a 60 year-old male clutching his chest: "I don't want to hear any more about your chest pains. Do you have any idea how many men your age come in here complaining of chest pains? Or, how often chest pains are misdiagnosed as heart-related? Chest pains can be caused by a number of benign medical conditions, so the odds are that yours are nothing serious. Besides, your chest pains are what got you admitted to the ER. Statistically speaking, it would be inappropriate for us to give them any weight in the diagnostic process. So, unless you have other symptoms to report, we'll be sending you home." (Everson & Faller, 2012, pp. 45–46)

We agree with the fundamental points these authors make about not disregarding useful indicators, but this has absolutely *nothing* to do with any position we hold or intended to convey about double-dipping and its negative consequences. Again, we regret the extent to which our description of the problem may have contributed to this disconnect, and we attempt to provide further clarification here.

To succinctly reiterate, the double-dipping argument states that once an indicator is used in the screening phase, it lacks additional *differentiating* value at the diagnostic phase. That is, if a variable is used to identify individuals who will be further assessed, then all individuals at the next level of assessment possess this same variable. All of the true positives and false positives in our smaller screened group now have the same characteristic; therefore, this characteristic is not of further—or incremental—utility in *differentiating* the true positives from the false positives. This does *not* imply that the indicator had no value in the first place, that it does not continue to be of value, or that it should not be referred to again for further diagnostic decisions.

For example, if 90% of individuals with a certain symptom have condition X, that indicator is obviously of considerable value. If we form a group of only those with this symptom, 90% will have condition X, with all of the implications this might have for diagnosis or treatment. But we should not conclude that *more than* 90% of these individuals have condition X because everyone in the group has the symptom nor use this exact same information to further alter likelihood estimates. Rather, to achieve greater certainty, we now seek other variables that, when combined with the first variable, further enhance accuracy. Even assuming we cannot find any such additional variables, we still possess this single, highly valuable diagnostic sign, and, although we would not alter the 90% probability estimate, this level of certainty may surely be of great value in guiding judgment and intervention. The risk, however, of double counting this symptom, especially when initial indicators are iffy and judgments are overly swayed by information that is entirely redundant and really should not change anything, is greater (or much greater) certainty than is warranted. Maintaining a greater sense of subjective confidence than is justified leads to various undesirable decision-making practices, all of which tend to decrease accuracy, including the underweighting of other variables that, ironically, may yield incremental validity (e.g., Faust & Ahern, 2011).

For illustrative purposes, suppose a mugging victim approaches police, describing the assailant as a "very tall man." Police apprehend several suspects—all quite tall—who were known to be in the area at the time of the crime and who have past convictions for theft or assault. A lineup is created, and the victim asked to identify the perpetrator. Here, the screening criterion—"very tall"—was used to identify a number of possible assailants. However, only one is truly the mugger (and identifying him as such would be a true positive) while the others in the lineup are not (and identifying one of them as such would be a false positive). All of the suspects in the lineup are very tall and, as such, height will not provide further help in separating the true positives from the false positives. We now wish to obtain additional variables that augment our information and provide differentiating value among this group; here, perhaps, a facial scar, tattoo, or distinct vocal tone. To assume it would be our position that no person could be charged for the crime because more than one potential criminal is very tall is not accurate at all.

Furthermore, this characteristic might be introduced at trial later in time and serve a useful function. The defense attorney may, for example, try to pin the crime on another suspect who happens to be five feet, two inches tall, at which point the prosecution may contend the victim originally identified the mugger as very tall. There is nothing in our double-dipping argument contending that the value of the diagnostic indicator cannot be carried forward to other situations or circumstances and applied to the extent it has utility. Rather, the problem we describe involves a failure to recognize the boundaries of a diagnostic sign or indicator's utility by mistakenly assuming (or acting as if) the sign possesses incremental value even after one has narrowed the group to those who share the sign. Our concern is double-dipping appears to be a common error with deleterious consequences.

To return to Everson and Faller's (2012) first example, we have no disagreement with a number of their points, including (a) chest pain is the screening criterion and resulted in the patient seeking further evaluation at the ER and (b) many benign conditions may cause chest pain, and, therefore, the patient may truly be having a heart attack (true positive) or a panic attack (false positive). Our point is that chest pain cannot help to further differentiate or better distinguish between those two groups (heart attacks and panic attacks) *at this point*, so what one seeks are additional valid predictors that can differentiate the two groups and augment the information we already have available. Blood enzyme tests or an EKG will serve just that purpose. However, if we are, say, in a rural setting and do not have an EKG or an enzyme panel readily available, this does not mean the original indicator— the chest pain—should be ignored. We did not and are not suggesting this in any way, shape, or form. In our chapters, we place great emphasis on the validity or utility of screening procedures, which would not make sense if we also take the position that those variables should be forgotten once one gets to the clinic for further evaluation. Whether addressing Everson and Faller's examples involving cardiology or sexual abuse, these same clarifying statements apply.

Everson and Faller (2012) contend that the double-dipping argument is problematic for two additional reasons: first, that a shift occurs between the screening and evaluation phase that transforms the role of abuse indicators, and, second, that diagnostic indicators "used at screening are often enhanced during the forensic evaluation phase by a process akin to separating wheat from chaff" (p. 65). We do not wish to enter into an argument over particulars here because we do not think they truly intersect with the principles we enumerate. The process Everson and Fuller describe—culling and refining, revisiting variables to find out additional information, clarifying reports or symptoms, and "consider[ing] the likely cause or meaning of the abuse indicator" (p. 66)—seems distinguishable from our proposal for avoiding double-dipping. If a process or procedure is implemented in the evaluation phase rendering a variable more definitive, then the variable's value changes and the new value should be incorporated into decision making. For example, if a "yes" to a certain question is initially somewhat tentative and further evaluation yields a more definitive answer with higher predictive value, then standing on the variable or its informational value changes; the variable then can and should be used in further decision making. If, for example, a predictor originally possessing 60% accuracy is further refined or clarified via additional evaluation and now achieves 80% accuracy, the use of the latter is not double-dipping because unique predictive information was added. What we do question here is whether procedures believed to change or enhance the predictive value of variables really do so. That is, do such transformations achieve the level of improvement assumed? When such procedures do not make any true change, then, to the extent falsely inflated beliefs alter decision making, they may take on the functional equivalent of double-dipping.

BAYESIAN ANALYSES

Finally, Lyon, Ahern, and Scurich (2012) critiqued our argument that some apparently valid measures may lead to increased error in judgment when applied under certain circumstances. We believe Lyon and colleagues make a number of worthwhile points and suggest that those less familiar with the critical importance of base rates in decision making read their cogent presentation. We agree with these authors' reminder that a Bayesian approach to decision making means adjusting the probability of an outcome or condition when new information is provided and, absent any other information, the starting probability is the base rate. The authors also describe the use of odds ratios to convey probabilities.

We believe there are few differences between our arguments and those of Lyon and colleagues (2012) on basic principles involving the application of base rates. As such, the extent of seeming disagreement rests largely at our feet. First, we discovered that one source of confusion originates in our use of odds ratios: at times, we report percentages as though they were odds ratios (e.g., in the appendix of Chapter 1, we incorrectly represent 75% as 3:4 rather than 3/4).

Second, our use of "accuracy" in this context promulgated confusion, likely because we took an expository shortcut that, given more usual presentations on this topic, was prone to misinterpretation. We agree with Lyon and colleagues (2012) that our definition of accuracy is nonstandard because it refers to both true-positive and true-negative rates. In such types of analyses, it is necessary to look at both the prior odds and the diagnosticity of methods then the end result when the two factors are combined. Depending on the prior odds or base rates, a method possessing validity (or intrinsic accuracy) may, nonetheless, produce more erroneous than correct positive identifications. For example, a carefully designed neuropsychological test might possess validity and hence, when applied to an overall group with a 50% frequency of brain damage, may be correct in classifying cases most of the time. Nevertheless, if the frequency of brain damage is very low in the group of interest—say, for example, 5%—most of the positive identifications of brain damage could be wrong. Similarly, in settings in which the base rate for sexual abuse is low, even valid (or "accurate") tests can be wrong more often than right in identifying positive cases. In our chapters (Faust, Bridges, & Ahern, 2009a, 2009b; Bridges, Faust, & Ahern, 2009), we use "accuracy" to refer to this latter type of circumstance (i.e., the end result when both base rates and the diagnosticity of methods are taken into account) in which case positive identifications may be less accurate than a coin toss. However, it would have been preferable to distinguish the accuracy of the test from its efficacy when the base rates are also taken into account and to not refer to positive identifications in isolation (but to also consider negative identifications).

Consequently, our comment about achieving an accuracy rate of 38%, or "worse than a coin toss," was potentially misleading, and the technically correct comparison is between the odds when including the test (3:5 odds the child was abused) and the original odds (1:5 odds the child was abused). Indeed, the latter comparison makes it evident that the decision maker moves from a position of being fairly certain a child was not abused to a more equivocal stance. Our use of the coin-toss comparison is meant to inform the reader that, under a low base rate condition, even a good indicator of abuse may still not leave us in a position to be anything other than "less certain" the child is not abused and not necessarily "more certain than uncertain" the child is abused. We also noted an error in the equation provided in the appendix of Chapter 1. We present a formula for determining odds of being sexually abused. However, we inadvertently left out a set of parentheses in the denominator term. The formula should read: $Pp_1/(Pp_1 + Qp_2)$.

On a final note, we wish to address Everson and Faller's (2012) argument indicating "the use of multiple indicators trumps the impact of base rates" (p. 56). The assumption that multiple indicators surpass base rates merits consideration; however, the author's analysis disregards redundancy of variables. In practice, complete or near orthogonality of variables is quite rare, especially if more than a few indicators are involved. As such, the boost in incremental validity from combined variables is often far less than might be assumed. In addition, one often approaches or reaches a ceiling in accuracy after a relatively small number of predictors are taken into account, particularly if one identifies the most valid and least redundant combination (Faust & Ahern, 2011). Furthermore, combining or adding weaker variables with stronger predictors can degrade accuracy. Thus, beliefs or assumptions about the value of multiple indicators need to be tested through formal scientific study: they may turn out to be correct or well off the mark based on the nature of the variables utilized. That multiple indicators will decidedly trump the use of base rates cannot be taken as a given.

More generally, there is often no reason to view base rates and tests or methods as opposing one another. Instead, they may frequently serve as data points or sources of information that can and should be properly combined to achieve better estimates of likelihood. This combination might sometimes yield highly informative if not stunning results (i.e., more false positive than valid positive identifications).

CONCLUSIONS

We would like to reiterate our appreciation, both for those commentators who offered their insights on our chapters and for the opportunity to further elucidate our ideas. The assessment of child sexual abuse is an issue of enormous weight and consequence, and the continued development and refinement of accurate methods and tools is of great importance. We look forward to the continued discussion of these issues and the continued growth of this field.

REFERENCES

Bridges, A. J., Faust, D., & Ahern, D. C. (2009). Methods for the identification of sexually abused children: Reframing the clinician's task and recognizing its disparity with research on indicators. In K. Kuehnle & M. Connell (Eds.), *The evaluation of child sexual abuse allegations: A comprehensive guide to assessment and testimony* (pp. 21–47). New York: Wiley.

Everson, M. D., & Faller, K. C. (2012). Base rates, multiple indicators, and comprehensive forensic evaluations: Why sexualized behavior still counts in assessments of child sexual abuse allegations. *Journal of Child Sexual Abuse, 21*(1), 45–71.

Faust, D., & Ahern, D. C. (2011). Clinical judgment and prediction. In D. Faust (Ed.), *Coping with psychiatric and psychological testimony* (6th ed., pp. 147–208). New York: Oxford University Press.

Faust, D., Bridges, A. J., & Ahern, D. C. (2009a). Methods for the identification of sexually abused children: Issues and needed features for abuse indicators. In K. Kuehnle & M. Connell (Eds.), *The evaluation of child sexual abuse allegations: A comprehensive guide to assessment and testimony* (pp. 3–19). New York: Wiley.

Faust, D., Bridges, A. J., & Ahern, D. C. (2009b). Methods for the identification of sexually abused children: Suggestions for clinical work and research. In K. Kuehnle & M. Connell (Eds.), *The evaluation of child sexual abuse allegations: A comprehensive guide to assessment and testimony* (pp 49–79). New York: Wiley.

Lyon, T. D., Ahern, E. C., & Scurich, N. (2012). Interviewing children versus tossing coins: Accurately assessing the diagnosticity of children's disclosures of abuse. *Journal of Child Sexual Abuse, 21*(1), 19–44.

AUTHOR NOTES

David C. Ahern, PhD, Alpert Medical School of Brown University, Providence, RI.

Ana J. Bridges, PhD, Department of Psychology, University of Arkansas, Fayetteville, AR.

David Faust, PhD, Department of Psychology, University of Rhode Island, Kingston, RI, and Alpert Medical School of Brown University, Providence, RI.

What Poole and Wolfe (2009) Actually Said: A Comment on Everson and Faller (2012)

DEBRA ANN POOLE
Central Michigan University, Mt. Pleasant, Michigan, USA

Everson and Faller's (2012) article on the significance of sexualized behavior in child sexual abuse assessments critiques a chapter by Poole and Wolfe (2009), but their objections assumed conclusions and practice implications that were not contained in that chapter. In this comment, I reiterate the value of educating adults about normative sexual and nonsexual behavior that could be misconstrued as symptoms of sexual abuse in some children, review key points from the chapter, and point out that Everson and Faller's critique supports the chapter's take-home messages (i.e., the importance of gathering information from multiple sources and the need to test alternative hypotheses for concerning behavior, consider the overall context of individual cases, and obtain independent verification of evidence).

Mark Everson and Kathleen Faller's (2012) article on the role of sexualized behavior in child sexual abuse (CSA) assessments critiques a chapter I wrote with Michelle Wolfe (2008), but the chapter they take issue with was not one that we wrote. Here I briefly address the origin of our review, its contents, and Everson and Faller's major points before explaining how their critique ironically supports our take-home message.

We wrote our chapter after Kathy Kuehnle and Mary Connell asked us to review normative sexual and nonsexual behavior that could be misconstrued as symptoms of sexual abuse in individual children when, in fact, the behavior had other origins (Kuehnle & Connell, 2009). Because another chapter would also discuss sexual behavior, Michelle Wolfe and I focused on frequent behaviors and parental complaints. We used a criterion by Friedrich and colleagues (1998) to select behaviors for a table on developmentally related sexual behaviors, and our guidelines consisted of basic developmental findings, a statement that knowledge of development can help evaluators craft hypotheses, and a lament regarding a gap in knowledge. We concluded the following:

> The task of evaluating children will always involve looking at how current behavior compares with past behavior, how recent issues in the family and at school may relate to troubling behavior, and what picture is conveyed by the overall intensity of symptoms, the number of related problems, and the expression of problem behavior across contexts. Finally, many children who are sexually abused show no behaviors that alarm or alert adults, so the absence of behavioral change cannot be taken as evidence that abuse has not occurred. (Poole & Wolfe, 2009)

In their critique, Everson and Faller (2012) repeatedly claim we argued "against the use of sexual behavior problems in the forensic process" (p. 52). On the contrary, we said that "children who have been sexually abused are more likely than nonabused children to show sexualized behavior" and that "age-inappropriate sexual behavior and knowledge have long been considered the most specific behavioral markers of sexual abuse" (Poole & Wolfe, 2009, p. 112). This, however, was not the focus of our chapter: our goal was to catalog behaviors that were so common that, depending on the context and other case features, an individual child demonstrating those behaviors may be more likely to be nonabused than abused. We hoped this information would be valuable to parents, would help evaluators adjust the nature of assessments for individual cases, and would increase the probability of appropriate referrals (e.g., so physicians could rule out medical issues that frequently cause some symptoms).

Inexplicably, Everson and Faller (2012) summarize our message as follows: "The diagnostic value of sexualized behavior in CSA assessments is overrated. Forensic evaluators who rely on sexualized behavior are likely to overestimate the strength of the evidence in support of abuse. This will lead to a large number of false allegations of sexual abuse being mistakenly substantiated as true" (p. 52). Actually, in our chapter we explained why normative information is useful (e.g., "information about normative behavior prevents evaluators from developing convictions that abuse occurred based on behavior that is unrelated or only weakly related to abuse"; Poole & Wolfe, 2009, p. 101), and we included basic information about the reliability (or lack thereof) of information obtained from only one caregiver, as well as some common pitfalls of human judgment. We did not, however, critique the current state of CSA evaluations or speculate about rates of false substantiations.

Everson and Faller (2012) continued with five specific points:

1. Poole and Wolfe said there is substantial evidence that sexual curiosity and sexual behavior is normal, even among very young children (see p. 52). We did say that. Their response that more intrusive sexual behavior was rare does not rebut us because we did not discuss low-frequency behavior.
2. Poole and Wolfe said that caregiver reports of child behavior problems including sexual behaviors are known to be unreliable, inaccurate, and often biased (see p. 53). We warned evaluators that caregivers' reports of children's behavioral changes, particularly internalizing behaviors (e.g., sadness, depression), are subject to biases (e.g., may reflect caregivers' own anxieties). We did not address the reliability of reports of sexual behavior.
3. Poole and Wolfe said there are no diagnostic behavior indicators of sexual abuse, including aberrant sexualized behavior, that occur in all or even most abused children, while being simultaneously absent in all nonabused children (see p. 53). We said it was "an error ... to assume that most children who show inappropriate sexual behavior were sexually abused," and we explained why this is (e.g., "The majority of sexual behavior occurs among nonabused children simply because sexual behavior is common and there are more nonabused than abused children" and "less than half of all children who are sexually abused display this type of behavior, and such behavior is also associated with family problems, physical abuse, total life stress, and psychiatric disturbances"; Poole & Wolfe, 2009, p. 112). Our statement that "sexual behavior is not as valid a marker of sexual abuse as once thought" (p. 112), in the context of a chapter on normative behavior, cautioned professionals against overreliance on a single high-frequency behavior that is not a strong indicator of abuse. Everson and Faller do not appear to disagree with this.
4. Poole and Wolfe said that research has shown that sexualized behavior in children may result from a number of sources other than sexual abuse (see p. 54). Everson and Faller said they "concur with Poole and Wolfe" and explained that "the consensus in the field of forensic CSA assessment is that the presence of developmentally inappropriate sexual behaviors is insufficient to support a conclusion of CSA" (p. 54).
5. Poole and Wolfe said that reported differences in the rates of sexualized behavior in abused and nonabused children are likely exaggerated because of sampling biases (see p. 54). We cautioned readers to not take prevalence estimates too literally, but we worry that Everson and Faller will confuse readers because they juxtaposed their own language. Specifically, we said that "reported differences in rates of sexualized behavior between sexually abused and nonabused groups are likely exaggerated because sexual behavior can trigger discovery of sexual abuse, and therefore samples of children with documented histories of sexual

abuse may include a disproportionate number of children who displayed inappropriate sexual behavior" (Poole & Wolfe, 2009, pp. 112–113). Everson and Faller summarized this by saying that "children who have been abused may be overrepresented among those children whose sexualized behavior is discovered, *even if abused and nonabused children do not actually differ overall in sexualized behavior*" (italics added; p. 55). This implied that we questioned whether sexual behavior is an indicator when we did not.

Everson and Faller's critique of our chapter actually endorses our take-home message. Their defense of the CHIC (comprehensive, hypothesis-testing, idiographic, corroborative) evaluation model emphasizes gathering information from a wide range of sources, testing alternative hypotheses for concerning behavior, considering the unique contexts of individual cases, and obtaining independent verification of substantive evidence—all recommendations that follow from the studies we reviewed.

Why is this perspective difficult to embody? Partly because the *conditionalization* of knowledge (knowing when and where specific knowledge is relevant) is characteristic of advanced expertise—expertise that takes many years and specific types of feedback to develop (see Bransford, Brown, & Cocking, 2000). In the field of sexual abuse evaluations, conditionalization involves such things as an awareness that statements made in response to open-ended questions are typically accurate when children have not been exposed to misinformation about touching experiences but that a number of factors significantly decrease the reliability of "spontaneous" reports. Conditionalization is also involved when practitioners realize that false allegation rates vary as a function of case characteristics and that rates of sexualized behavior vary across families with different characteristics and recent experiences.

In the introduction to the special issue, Faller and Everson (2012) lament a clinician's lack of expertise and place blame for the fact that the clinician ignored signs of abuse partly on our chapter:

> She also had read Poole and Wolfe's (2009) chapter that points out that there are no sexual behaviors that are found only in sexually abused children. Therefore, she did not put a great deal of weight on the mother's digital penetration and finger licking report. (p. 8)

Faller and Everson (2012) make no mention of the fact that we acknowledged the indicator status of sexual behavior, that we said that "unusual and age-inappropriate behavior warrants investigation to determine where children are getting their knowledge" (p. 113), and that we wrote our chapter to precede another on the continuum of children's sexual behavior—a chapter which said that "aberrant sexual behavior is considered the most explicit effect and one of the most treatment-resistant symptoms associated with sexual abuse" (Gurley, Kuehnle, & Kirkpatrick, 2009, p. 130).

To conclude, the real controversy lies not in opinions about sexual behavior but in opinions about the ways some practitioners are exploring abuse suspicions (e.g., Faller and I do not agree on the appropriateness of some assessment techniques for some types of cases). But this is not an issue we addressed in Kuehnle and Connell (2009), so I am left wondering what Everson and Faller accomplished by misrepresenting the practice implications of an accurate chapter that supports their goal of informed approaches for protecting children and families.

REFERENCES

Bransford, J. D., Brown, A. L., & Cocking, R. R. (Eds.). (2000). *How people learn: Brain, mind, experience, and school* (expanded edition). Washington, DC: National Academy Press. Retrieved from http://www.nap.edu/openbook.php?isbn=0309070368

Everson, M. D., & Faller, K. C. (2012). Base rates, multiple indicators, and comprehensive forensic evaluations: Why sexualized behavior still counts in assessments of child sexual abuse allegations. *Journal of Child Sexual Abuse*, *21*(1), 45–71.

Faller, K. C., & Everson, M. D. (2012). Contested issues in the evaluation of child sexual abuse allegations: Why consensus on best practice remains elusive. *Journal of Child Sexual Abuse*, *21*, 3–18.

Friedrich, W. N., Fisher, J., Broughton, D., Houston, M., & Safran, C. R. (1998). Normative sexual behavior in children: A contemporary sample. *Pediatrics*, *101*, E9.

Gurley, J., Kuehnle, K., & Kirkpatrick, H. D. (2009). The continuum of children's sexual behavior: Discriminative categories and the need for public policy change. In K. Kuehnle & M. Connell (Eds.), *The evaluation of child sexual abuse allegations* (pp. 129–150). New York: Wiley.

Kuehnle, K., & Connell, M. (Eds.). (2009). *The evaluation of child sexual abuse allegations: A comprehensive guide to assessment and testimony* (pp. 101–128). New York: Wiley.

Poole, D. A., & Wolfe, M. S. (2009). Child development: Normative sexual and nonsexual behaviors that may be confused with symptoms of sexual abuse. In K. Kuehnle & M. Connell (Eds.), *The evaluation of child sexual abuse allegations: A comprehensive guide to assessment and testimony* (pp. 101–128). New York: Wiley.

AUTHOR NOTE

Debra Ann Poole, Department of Psychology, Central Michigan University, Mt. Pleasant, Michigan.

Index

Note: Page numbers in *italic* type refer to tables

accreditation 67
accuracy 45–8, 74, 82, 151–2; allegation 151–2; case decision-making 44–60; definition 22–3; seventy-five percent argument 22–4; substantiation decisions 45–6; versus coin toss 22–4, 163
Ahern, D.: Bridges, A. and Faust, D. 82–3, 133–5, 156–65
Ahern, E.: Scurich, N. and Lyon, T. 11, 18–43, 162
aids, interviewing 115–19; dolls 25–8, 49–51, 115–16; drawings 115–17; media 115
alcoholism 109
Aldridge, J.: *et al* 116
allegation 151–2
Aman, C.: and Goodman, G. 28
ambiguity 56–8, *57*; minimal 56–7; moderate 56–7; substantial 56–7
American Association for Marriage and Family Therapy (AAMFT) 139
American Bar Association (ABA) 139
American Professional Association on the Abuse of Children (APSAC) 140; *Psychological Evaluation of Suspected Abuse in Children Guidelines* 140
American Prosecutors Research Institute (APRI) 115; *Finding Words* 115
American Psychological Association (APA) 139
anal touch 27
assessment techniques 5; double-dipping 133–5, 156–62; hypotheticals as literal 157–9; identification methods 156–65; judgemental accuracy 29; and objectivity 3, *see also* indicators
attorneys/prosecutors 54, 67, 68, 72–4
Australia: Family Court 120–1

Bala, N.: and Trocme, N. 121
base rates 20, 91–9, 163; Bayesian approach 93–7; case example 93; disparity 92; and sampling biases 90–1, 168
Bayesian Theorem 5, 11, 18, 37, 91–101, 156–7, 162–4; approach 19–20; case example 93–9; and diagnosticity 18, 37–8; evidence of abuse

assessment 20–2; simplified 97–9, *98*; traditional 93–7, *95*
behavior changes 94–8, 157–8; moods 96; self-destructive 109, *see also* sexual behaviors
Bell, L. 75
best practice consensus 2–17; sensitivity vs specificity 5–12
brain size/IQ 109
Bridges, A.: *et al* 99; Faust, D. and Ahern, D. 82–3, 133–5, 156–65
Briere, J.: and Elliott, D. 111, 121
Brown, D.: and Lamb, M. 19, 114–15, 118
Brown, T.: *et al* 122
Browne, A.: and Finkelhor, D. 83–5
Bruck, M.: and Ceci, S. 27–8; *et al* 26–7

caregivers 89, 141; non-offending 73, 112
case ambiguity degree 56
case decision-making 44–62, 87–8; accuracy and objectivity 44–60; ambiguity 56; case material 48–9; criteria 51; demographic characteristics 54; design features 50–3; established practice 45–6; reliability 47–50, *49*; three-part rebuttal 46–58; variation impacts 53–8
case summaries 55–6
Ceci, S.: and Bruck, M. 27–8
CHIC evaluation model 11, 86–90, 100–3, 169; comprehensive 11, 86; corroborative 11, 87–8; duplicative use of variables 100; hypothesis-testing 11, 87; idiographic 11, 87–8; screening process 100
Child Behavior Checklist (CBCL) 7, 101
child forensic evaluators (CFE) 54
child forensic interviewers (CFI) 54
child protection professionals 65–7, 75
Child Protective Services (CPS) 7–8, 50, 86, 93; case example 93–7; Denver 53; effectiveness 75; investigators 8–9; practice 51–2, 59; workers 54
Child Sexual Behavior Inventory (CSBI) 11, 84, 88–9, 101
Children's Advocacy Centers (CACs) 3, 8–12, 137–43, 148; assessment objectivity 3; case

INDEX

review 70; child assent 73; as coordinators 64; forensic interviewer 69–70; investigation teams 68–9; investigation vs treatment distinction 149–50; MDTs 68; mental health professionals' involvement 70–1, 137–43; National (Huntsville, Alabama) 69, 74–6, 113–15, 146; primary goals 138; rights promotion 78; role conflict 63–80, 137–42; standard practice 69; surveys 77; types of professionals 67

Clark, C. 7

clinician perceptions 76; among clients/public 76–7

clothes off question 27–8

cognitive interview (CI): five-stage 118–19

Cohen's kappa coefficients 47

comprehensive forensic evaluation (CFE) model 48; CHIC 86–8; and interviewing 108–23; and sexualized behavior assessments 81–103

Connell, M. 64–71, 74–7, 138–41, 148–55; and Kuehnle, K. 2–13, 19, 46, 82, 120, 130–5, 152, 166, 170

Cordisco-Steele, L.: Nelson-Gardell, D. and Faller, K. 115

Cornerhouse RATAC 116

Cramer, R. (Bud) 74

criminal justice 12, 64–5, 69, 75, 137; truth-seeking and prosecuting 66–9

Cross, T.: *et al* 12, 63–80, 144–6, 148–55; Jones, P. and Walsh, L. 64, 138

Cross, W.: and Fine, J. 64

curiosity 88–9, 168

custody disputes 13; and allegations 120–2; neglect 120; risk and safety 122

decision-making *see* case decision-making

Denver Child Protective Services (CPS) 53

depression 109; women with CSA history 109–10

developmental disabilities 117

developmental screening 115

Developmentally Related Sexual Behaviors (DRSB) 89

DeVoe, E.: and Faller, K. 121

diagnosticity 18–43, 22; analysis differences 35–6; coin toss vs accuracy tests 22–4, 163; criteria 89; disclosure statements 18–38; genital touch disclosure 25–8; interview methods 30–5; lack of 89; unrealistic assumptions and likelihood 24–5

DiPietro, E.: *et al* 111

disclosure 13, 100, 109, 154; active 13; child's statement 3, 18–38; and corroborative evidence 96–7; definition restriction 96–7; diagnosticity 18–43; false 36; genital touch 25–8; intentionally false 121; likelihood ratio 21; motivational factors 114; potential redundancy 29–30; recantation rate 114; true 36; verbal 115

disputes: custody 13, 120–2

dissociative identity disorder (DID) 89; and sexual abuse relationship 90

DNA testing 36

dolls and sexual play 25, 115–16; genital touch disclosure 25–8; interviews 49–51

double-dipping 133–5, 156–62; argument flaw 100; case example 100; and differentiation 99, 158–60; disclosure potential redundancy 29–30; screening process 100; variables 161–3

drawings 115–17

drug dependence 109

Dubowitz, H.: *et al* 111

Elliott, D.: and Briere, J. 111, 121

enforcement officers 54, 67

ethical issues 112; code 139

Evaluation of Child Sexual Abuse Allegations (Kuehnle and Connell) 2–13, 46; and double-dipping 133–5; partial disagreement 130–5

Everson, M.: *et al* 12, 44–62; and Faller, K. 2–17, 81–107, 114, 131, 135, 158–63, 166–70

evidence 23; corroborating/hard 9–11, 46, 110–11, 130–3; credible 51; physical 109; probative 111; psychosocial 44–60; soft 44, 132–3; weak 23

expert witness testimony 5, 71, 130–1

exposure types 86

Extended Forensic Evaluation (EFE) 152–4

Faller, K. 59, 86, 122; Cordisco-Steele, L. and Nelson-Gardell, D. 115; and DeVoe, E. 121; and Everson, M. 2–17, 81–107, 114, 131, 135, 158–63, 166–70; Michigan clinic 121; and Palusci, V. 66, 74

false accusations 8, 13; risk 59–60

false negatives 3, 110–13; errors 3–4; potential 111

false positives 3, 13, 110–13, 160; errors 3–4

Family Court of Australia 120–1

Faust, D. 88, 92; Ahern, D. and Bridges, A. 82–3, 133–5, 156–65; *et al* 7, 11, 19, 23–4, 29, 89, 92–8, 102

field-relevant research 108–28; CSA impacts 109–10; custody dispute allegations 120–2; developmental screening 115; false positives/negatives 110–13; future directions and approaches 113; interview aids/manners 115–19; interview techniques/protocols 114–15; peer review and supervision 119–20

Fine, J. 64, 138, 144–6, 148–55; and Cross, W. 64

Finkelhor, D.: and Browne, A. 83–5

Finlayson, L.: and Koocher, G. 47, 51

Finnila, K.: *et al* 27

Fisher, R.: and Geiselman, R. 118

INDEX

five-stage cognitive interview (CI) 118–19; probed recall 119
forensic methodology 3; evaluations 9, 81–103; structured format 10; validity 3, *see also* interview techniques
forensic neutrality 148–55; and EFE 152–4; therapist assisting prosecution 151–2
Friedrich, W. 11, 84, 89–90; behavior norms 93, 167
Friend, C. 137–43

Geiselman, R.: and Fisher, R. 118
genital touch disclosure 25–8; occurrences 33
Goldstein, S. 144–7
Goodman, G.: and Aman, C. 28
guilt 94
Guyer, M.: Kalter, N. and Horner, T. 47

hard evidence 9–11, 46, 110–11, 130–3
Heger, A.: *et al* 25
Herman, S. 11–12, 19, 44–6, 112–13; analysis differences 35–6; false dichotomy and related foibles 131–3; *Forensic Child Sexual Abuse Evaluations* 131–3; reliability argument 47–50, 58–60
Hershkowitz, I. 116; *et al* 35–7, 47–8; and Terner, A. 114
HIV/AIDS 109
Horner, T.: *et al* 47, 50; Guyer, M. and Kalter, N. 47

identity 89, 90
Illinois Supreme Court 132
impact: of CSA 109–12
In re A.P. (1997) 132
In re Nicole V (1987) 130
indicators 10, 97, 161; abuse 7, 11, 92; Bayesian approach 93–9, 95, 98; behavior changes 3, 94–7; and comprehensive forensic evaluations 81–103; diagnostic value 11, 168; evaluation-level 101–2; multiple 95; non-redundant 96–8; population base rates 91–9; probability 10; screening-level 101; sexual abuse 89–90; survey-level 101
institutional review board (IRB) 49
intentionality 32–3
interview: Ten Step 35–7
interview techniques 5, 18; additional protocols 117–19; aids 115–19; and allegations in custody dispute context 120–2; children with developmental disabilities 117; developmental screening 115; disclosure diagnosticity increase 30–5; false negatives 110–13; false positives 110–11; field-relevant research 13, 108–23; five-stage cognitive (CI) 118–19; future directions and approaches 113; and guidelines 115; interviewer manner 119; misleading questions 28; narrative elaboration (NET) 118; peer review and supervision 119–20; reluctant/recanting children 114–15; repeated/extended protocols 114–15; research 114–15; and sexual abuse impact 109–10; toolkit 117–18
investigation teams 68–9; law enforcement 94; medical/mental health professionals 68–9; prosecutors 68, 72–4; and therapeutic staff proximity 76; victim witness advocates 68, *see also* multidisciplinary teams
investigation vs treatment distinction 149–50
IQ/brain size 109
Israel 46; child abuse investigators 46; and NICHD protocol 114, 119–20

Jackson, H.: and Nuttall, R. 47
Jensen, J.: *et al* 75; Wescoe, S. and Realmuto, G. 47
Jones, P.: Walsh, L. and Cross, T. 64, 138, 144–6, 148–55
Journal of Child Sexual Abuse (Faller and Everson) 131, 135
judgments: professional *see* reliability of professional judgments

Kalter, N.: Horner, T. and Guyer, M. 47
Katz, C. 116
Kimbrough-Melton, R.: and Melton, G. 12, 64–77, 138–9, 145, 148–9, 154
Koch, G.: and Landis, R. 57
Kolbo, J.: and Strong, E. 75
Koocher, G.: and Finlayson, L. 47, 51
Kuehnle, K. 88; and Connell, M. 2–13, 19, 46, 82, 120, 130–5, 152, 166, 170

La Rooy, D.: Lamb, M. and Pipe, M. 114
Lamb, M.: and Brown, D. 19, 114–15, 118; Pipe, M. and La Rooy, D. 114
Lamb, T.: *et al* 113, 117
Landis, R.: and Koch, G. 57
law enforcement 94
legal issues 5, 130; accuracy of allegation 151–2; expert testimony 130–1; and hard evidence 130–3; therapist assisting prosecution 151–2; and truth 10
Leith, A. 72
likelihood 20; disclosure 21, 38; guidelines 86; percentage 19–20; ratio 20–2, 91–2, 95–101; unrealistic assumptions 24–5
Limber, S.: and Melton, G. 73
Lyon, T. 35; Ahern, E. and Scurich, N. 11, 18–43, 162; *et al* 99, 113

McGraw, J.: and Smith, H. 47, 50
McMartin Preschool case (1980s) 5
Martin, A.: and Schum, D. 30
masturbation: excessive 101–2

INDEX

media aids 115
medical health professionals 54, 67–72
Melton, G.: and Kimbrough-Melton, R. 12, 64–77, 138–9, 145, 148–9, 154; and Limber, S. 73
memory 5
mental health professionals 12, 54, 67–72, 137–40; and extended forensic evaluation (EFE) 152–4; as forensic interviewers 72; investigation vs treatment distinction 149–50; involvement in CACs 70–1, 137–43; objectives 12; as prosecutorial investigators 72–4; role boundary clarification 140, 148–54; role conflict 12, 63–80, 137–42
mock evaluation 55
moods 96
multidisciplinary team (MDT) 9, 68, 72–8; boundary clarification 148–54; and role conflict 68, 144–6
Myers, J. 5, 130–6

narrative elaboration technique (NET) 118
National Alliance on Mental Illness (NAMI) 139; code of ethics 139
National Association of Social Workers (NASW) 139
National Child Traumatic Stress Network (NCTSN) 64, 141
National Children's Alliance (NCA) 12, 67, 78, 138, 141; Standards for Accredited Members Revised (2011) 148; Standards Committee 64, 70–2
National Institutes of Child Health and Human Development (NICHD) 8, 108; interviewer manner 119; Investigative Interview Protocol 5, 8–9, 13, 19, 34–7, 113–18, 123; modifications 115; sequential questioning strategy 117
negative rate 23; false 110–13; true 23
neglect 120
Nelson-Gardell, D.: Faller, K. and Cordisco-Steele, L. 115
New York Court of Appeals 130
NJP (no judgment possible) category/case decisions 53; Exclusion of Undecided/indeterminate 57–8
no fault 122; and no risk 122
nomothetic methodology 87–8
non-offending caregivers 73
normative child development 5; sexual behavior 5
Nuttall, R.: and Jackson, H. 47

Oates, R.: et al 53
Office of Juvenile Justice and Delinquency Prevention (OJJDP) 142
Olafson, E. 13, 108–28
operationalization 56

Palusci, V.: and Faller, K. 66, 74
peer review: and supervision 119–20
Pennsylvania vs Ritchie case (1987) 130
Pipe, M.: La Rooy, D. and Lamb, M. 114
polyvictimization 109
Poole, D. 166–70; and Wolfe, M. 7, 11, 82–3, 88–91, 166–70
positive rate 22; false 22–3, 27–8, 110–11; true 22–3
Post-Traumatic Stress Disorder (PTSD) 101, 109
privacy protection 73
probability 10–11, 18–19, 94, 160; indicators 10, 95–7; posterior 97; prior 20, 24
probable cause 51
professionals 54, 68–71; attorneys/prosecutors 54, 67, 68, 72–4; child forensic evaluators (CFE) 54; child forensic interviewers (CFI) 54; child protection 65–7, 75; CPS workers 54; enforcement officers 54, 67; medical health 54, 67–72; victim advocacy 67; within CACs 67, *see also* mental health professionals; reliability of professional judgments
prosecution 67; affiliated facilities and employment 76–7; investigation teams 68–9; and mental health professionals 72–4; therapist assisting 151–2; truth-seeking 74–5; versus therapeutic model 74–5
prosecutors 54, 67, 68, 72–4
protocol criticisms 6–11; case study 6–11
psychologist roles 5
public health 122–3; unrecognised abuse 122

questions 30–5; and free recall reports 31; narrative practice 31; open-ended 30–1; placebic 32; source monitoring 34; wh- 30; what happened next 33, *see also* interview techniques

rape 109
Realmuto, G.: et al 49; Jensen, J. and Wescoe, S. 47
Record Review Exercise 55
reforms 45, 59; current practice 46
reinforcement 31–2; noncontingent 31–2
reliability of professional judgements 44–62; ambiguity 51; case information comprehensive vs narrow range 51; decision exercises 55; decision-making criteria provision 52–3; demographic characteristics 54; design features 50–8; established practice 45–6; findings 57–8; no judgement possible cases 53; prior research examination 47–50; protocol-by-case combinations 57–8; published studies summary 49; studies 52–3; substantiated (definition) 51–2, 56, 58–60; unsubstantiated (definition) 52; variations impacts 53–8, 57
reluctant/recanting children 114–15

INDEX

risk 122; false accusations 59–60
role conflict 3, 12, 144–6; boundary research 77–8; in CACs 63–80, 137–42; concerns 65–7, 71–7; consensus 152; consequences 65–6; inherent 75–6; in MDTs 68, 144–6; and mental health professionals 63–80, 137–42; mental health professionals 12, 63–80, 137–42; prosecution-affiliated facility employment 76–7; truth-seeking and prosecution 74–5

safety 122
sampling biases 90–1, 168
Saywitz, K.: *et al* 26–7, 118
Schum, D.: and Martin, A. 30
screening: developmental 115; methods 24–5, 160; sexual behaviors 85
Scurich, N.: Lyon, T. and Ahern, E. 11, 18–43, 162
self-destructive behavior changes 109
sensitivity 4, 12, 108; and specificity 5–12
Sexual Abuse Specific Items (SASI) 89
sexual behaviors 5, 81–107, 166–70; Bayesian approach 93–9; caregiver reports 89; case examples 93; and CHIC 86–8; curiosity 88–9, 168; diagnostic indicators 89–90, 99–102, 168–9; diagnostic value concerns 88–102, 167; misinterpretation/distortion 91; multiple roles 85–6; non-abuse origins 94; population base rates 7, 91–9; rates in abused and non-abused children 90–1; sampling biases 90–1; screening 85; and sexual abuse link 83–5; sources 90, 168; unwarranted use 82
Shumaker, K. 47
Smith, H.: and McGraw, J. 47, 50
specificity-over-sensitivity 4, 5–12, 82, 108
spillover effect 138
Stepwise Interview 113
Sternberg, K.: *et al* 31
Steward, M.: *et al* 26
Stone, Sam 34
Strong, E.: and Kolbo, J. 75
substantiation 45–6; decisions 45–6; definition 51–2, 56–7, 56; study design features 55–8

suggestibility 5–7, 27–9; and actual experiences 34
suspicion 24; and unrealistic assumptions 24–5

Teacher Report Forms 7
Ten-Step interview 35–7
Terner, A.: and Hershkowitz, I. 114
testimony 5; expert 5
therapeutic advocacy 11–12, 148–55; boundaries 78; clinician perceptions 76–7; collegial review goals 154; investigation and treatment distinction 149–50; service delivery 78
therapeutic role/techniques 145–6
threats 94
touching: genital 25–8, 33
trauma burden 83, 101; child's experiences 84–5; mechanisms 83–4
Trauma-Focused Cognitive Behavioral Therapy (TFCBT) 112
Trocme, N.: and Bala, N. 121
truth 10, 74–5

unrecognised abuse 122

validity 3, 35; case-decision making 45–7, 54–5; ecological 48; judgements 35; rating 50, 57–8; vs false cases 45, *see also* reliability
victim advocacy professionals 67
video recordings 49

Walsh, L.: Cross, T. and Jones, P. 64, 138, 144–6, 148–55
Wescoe, S.: Realmuto, G. and Jensen, J. 47
witness testimony: expert 5, 71, 130–1
Wolfe, M.: and Poole, D. 7, 11, 82–3, 88–91, 166–70
Wood, J. 21

Yuille, J. 113; Stepwise Interview 113